THE
WeLL-ResTed *W*oman

60 Soothing Suggestions
for Getting a Good Night's Sleep

Janet Kinosian

CONARI PRESS

Cover Photography: © Paul Vozdic/The Image Bank
Cover Design: Claudia Smelser
Book Design: Maxine Ressler
Author Photo: Levon Parian

Library of Congress Cataloging-in-Publication Data

Kinosian, Janet.
The well-rested woman : 60 soothing suggestions for getting a good
night's sleep / Janet Kinosian.
p. cm.
Includes bibliographical references.
ISBN 1-57324-813-4
1. Sleep. 2. Insomnia. 3. Women--Health and hygiene. I. Title.
RA786 .K56 2002
616.8'498'082--dc21
2002009407

Printed in Canada on recycled paper.

02   03   04   05   TC   10   9   8   7   6   5   4   3   2   1

For my parents,
who sang me endless perfect lullabies.
To M. E., S. A., N. P., H. T. & L. A.
and all my child dreamers yet to come.
In memory of my father, *with love*
who sleeps now in rarer air.

⌑⋘∾⌑

Sleep, my love, let my sleep
fall to me in prayer,
and as we were on earth,
so let us remain.
—GABRIELA MISTRAL

All I want is to sleep, long and deep,
the way a happy woman sleeps.
—ROSARIO CASTELLANOS

Sand-clock moon.
The night empties out,
the hour is lit.
—OCTAVIO PAZ

THE WELL-RESTED WOMAN

DISCLAIMER:

This book is not a substitute for the personal care and
medical advice of your physician. It should be used only
under the supervision and/or monitoring of your doctor or
other health-care professional to help with your sleep
difficulties. Do not take any medication, supplement, or
herb, or pursue any medical activity referenced in this
book without the permission of your doctor. If you are
taking prescription medications, notify your physician
about any new treatment, and do not take yourself off
any medicines or start supplementation without the supervision of your doctor.

PREFACE

...she slept the world.
—RAINER MARIA RILKE

WHEN I WAS A CHILD, I SLEPT SOUNDLY, dreamt sweetly, and awoke triumphantly. Back then, sleep was pure pleasure—as well as something I was good at—and each morning I took myself away from something luxurious, soft, and intoxicating. Somehow, as an adult, the whole sleep experience got badly fractured; many of the women I talk to say the same. What ever happened to those dreamy nights when we slept deeply, when we didn't wake up at 2 A.M. wondering what other sad soul might be awake at this odd hour? Where did all the peaceful slumber go?

I'm not an M.D., a Ph.D., nor a director of a sleep clinic. I am, however, a female insomnia sufferer who searched hard and ultimately found a good measure of peaceful sleep. I've spent the better part of fifteen years learning about sleep—from a layperson's point of view—and what to do and not do to help get a better night's rest. This is a book of sleep solutions shared with my sisters-in-sleeplessness, and any woman who simply desires better, more peaceful slumber. Like most good advice, the suggestions are not earth shattering. In fact, you've probably heard some of them before. But now is the time to truly *hear* them, use them as a blueprint, a way to teach and train yourself to naturally move into a place of better rest.

The Well-Rested Woman: 60 Soothing Suggestions for Getting a Good Night's Sleep is designed to help you, a woman, cultivate the seeds of better sleep. On a daily basis. One need not be a classic insomniac to benefit from some great tips for the often difficult task of getting a rejuvenating night's sleep. Take the book an essay at a time, flip through the pages, mull it over, read it straight through; however you use it, the wish is that better sleep will bring you expanded energy, spilling over and infusing your life.

The first two chapters, "What Is Sleep? Order and Disorder" and "Women and Sleep: Special Issues," give you straightforward factual information on sleep—what it is, what is its function, and what can go wrong—and information pertinent to women—how our hormones and reproductive system affect our sleep. The book's main feature—sixty fun and informative essays on sleep—offers scores of sleep solutions. Sectioned into six main categories, each highlights your sleep from a different vantage point. "Creating the Right Environment" offers suggestions to help transform your bedroom into a sleep oasis. "De-stressing the Mind," "Fine-Tuning the Body," and "Soothing the Soul" give you lovely, concrete ideas for the all-important task of de-stressing and preparing your body, mind, and soul for a better night's rest. "Sleep Hazards" lists things to avoid or watch out for, what I call "sleep stealers." Finally, the last chapter, "If You Need More Help," discusses further resources that can help with those sleepless nights.

I offer this book of sleep wisdom not within the impermeable boundaries of science, but, as Emily Dickinson would say, "from my certain slant of light." In it, take solace, serenity, succor, and some new secrets. And, of course, sweetest sleep.

Janet Kinosian

Los Angeles 2002

In Lumine Tuo Uidebimis Lumen
In Thy Light we shall see Light

CHAPTER 1

WHAT IS SLEEP?

ORDER AND DISORDER

If sleep does not secure an
absolutely vital function, then it is the
biggest mistake the evolutionary
process ever made.

—DR. ALLAN RECHTSCHAFFEN,
UNIVERSITY OF CHICAGO

I T'S NO SECRET THAT WOMEN TODAY ARE IN DIRE need of some restful nights. Modern life seems to conspire in subtle and not so subtle ways to lop off precious hours of sleep from many women's lives. You may wonder, Am I getting enough sleep? Probably not, if you work, run a household, go to school full time, supervise your family's lives, or simply make time just for yourself among the schedules you're juggling.

Even if you do think you're getting the amount of sleep you should, you may wonder why you feel so tired and unrefreshed much of the time. This is not surprising. More than *half of the women* surveyed in a recent National Sleep Foundation Women and Sleep Poll reported insomnia symptoms sometime during every month. Various studies and polls indicate that nearly *30 million American women* claim they long every day for a good night's sleep.

And despite what we sometimes think, a good night's sleep isn't a rare and exotic experience that occurs on high mountain tops and then only for those lucky enough to find it. Good sleep is an innate biological need—a need the body makes sure it fulfills, even with only a few healthy sleep habits.

In evolutionary terms, it was only minutes ago that science took notice of what happens when someone closes their eyes. Before the 1950s—when medicine first started unraveling the sleeping brain's mysteries—sleep was seen as a physiological, unmysterious, and natural daily happening, a true nonevent (it was only in 1996 that the American Medical Association recognized sleep medicine as a secondary specialty). Until the early '90s, women were often excluded from sleep studies because it was believed that their hormones would skew data. So women don't have a strong scientific history of help with sleep difficulties: health-care providers, medical information, and general self-help books didn't address the problem.

Much of this is changing, thankfully, and sleep researchers are beginning to study female sleep patterns and how they change over the course of a woman's life. Factors such as hormones, age, fertility, work, children, health, and lifestyle all affect your sleep, as do physical syndromes such as depression and pain, which affect women more than men. As the studies continue, you can look forward to more solid information on what's going on inside your body as you sleep, and how best to take advantage of the hours you do sleep.

The good news: A woman's sleep structure is fundamentally the same as a man's, but women have some distinct advantages. First, we experience more slow-wave or deep sleep, also called *stage 3 and 4 sleep,* throughout our lives.

Slow-wave deep sleep is the most restorative sleep level. In addition, our sleep systems age more slowly than do men's: while the amount of male slow-wave sleep diminishes after age twenty, female deep sleep has a slower decline, beginning after age thirty.

So if you hold the evolutionary gene for more restorative, deep sleep, why then do you not feel more deeply restored when you awake in the morning? If you guessed that modern lifestyle plays a role, that's a good guess. No longer is "Early to bed and early to rise" a guarantee of being well rested. To help find that good rest, take a brief look at what sleep is and what physical purpose it serves, what sleep disorders are and how you can deal with them.

WHY DO WE SLEEP?

Sleep research specialists still don't know exactly why we sleep, and medicine has not yet given us a central reason or function for it, though a variety of intriguing theories about sleep exist. We sleep to restore, rest, and repair vital physiological functions; to help activate the immune system; to program information and memory. One theory holds that sleep evolved as a means to remove our distant ancestors from harm and keep them safe during the dark hours of night.

Just how many hours of sleep do you need? Many people believe the traditional eight to be the most healthful number, yet most researchers claim this is myth. They believe you need only the number of sleep hours that make you feel consistently refreshed in the morning and fully alert during the day: if that number is five, then that's your physiological preference. You alone decide how much sleep your body needs. That nightly amount of needed sleep remains amazingly constant over a lifetime.

Whatever the biological reasons for sleep, we spend approximately a third of our lives in this state. For the average seventy-five-year-old, that means about twenty-three years of life spent sleeping.

THE STRUCTURE OF SLEEP

To understand sleep difficulties and disorders, it's important to understand sleep's two main stages: non-rapid eye movement sleep (NREM) and rapid eye movement sleep (REM) sleep.

NREM SLEEP

Non-rapid eye movement sleep is a four-stage cycle:

Stage 1 is the drowsy, relaxed, intermediary stage between waking and sleep. You are, in fact, half-awake, half-asleep, and your waking beta brain waves modulate to slower alpha and theta waves. Your body becomes more relaxed, but you're very easily awakened from this stage.

After several minutes in stage 1, you enter *stage 2* sleep. Your brain waves travel more slowly, intermittently mixing with what sleep researchers call "sleep spindles"; your breathing and heart rate stabilize, your muscles relax. Researchers use the first onset of a sleep spindle in an EEG (electroencephalogram) to mark the actual onset of sleep. It's still easy to awaken from this stage.

Stage 3 sleep produces slower theta waves and even slower delta waves. Your breathing slows, your heart rate slows more, and muscles become extremely relaxed. Most people reach this stage within 30 minutes after falling asleep. In this sleep stage the body releases growth hormone and regenerates, restores, and repairs organs and tissues. If awakened, you'll feel quite groggy.

Slow delta waves dominate *stage 4* sleep, the deepest sleep stage. This is the stage of sleep you must enter in order to feel rejuvenated and well rested. It's very difficult to awaken someone from this stage of sleep; if you are awakened, you'll feel groggy, even disoriented. Stage 4 is reached about an hour after falling asleep, and it's by far the most important sleep stage.

REM SLEEP

After the 90 minutes or so it takes to cycle through all four stages, you enter *rapid eye movement* sleep, a dream state that recurs every 70-90 minutes, lengthening throughout the night. Nearly 80 percent of dreams occur during REM sleep; your eyes dart back and forth as if you were watching a dream video screen, yet your body is incapable of muscular activity, so you can't act out your dreams. Meanwhile, heart and respiratory rates may speed up, and rapid brain waves, similar to those of a near-awake brain, occur.

After your first REM period, you awaken for a second or two—though you probably never notice it—and then cycle back through stages 2, 3, and 4 again, before entering another REM phase. Most deep stage 3 and 4 sleep occurs during the early part of the night; the REM periods lengthen so that your final one, just before you awaken, can last between 30 minutes and 1 hour. A good sleeper cycles through four to six of these cycles. It's quite normal to awaken briefly for a few seconds as you shift from stage to stage; most sleepers don't recall waking up.

WHAT ARE SLEEP DISORDERS?

It's no surprise that sleep disorders are common, what with all the intricate physical interactions necessary for a good night's sleep. What is surprising is how many disorders have already been cataloged—about seventy-five—yet millions of women still shrug off sleepless nights as simple insomnia. That's only partly true. Sleep troubles have many names and symptoms, and many possible solutions.

And while there are effective treatments for many of these sleep disorders, it's a safe bet that neither you nor your health-care provider knows the target symptoms for your particular disorder. Studies routinely indicate that only 3-5 percent of all people with sleep problems ask their doctors for help. And since sleep medicine is not currently taught in medical school, you're probably on your own when it comes to recognizing your symptoms and learning about your own sleep disorder.

As I'm not a trained sleep specialist, the following information on sleep disorders is culled from numerous interviews and topical resources, many of which are also available to you (see Resources).

TYPES OF SLEEP DISORDERS

Sleep disorders are grouped into two main categories: dyssomnia and parasomnias. *Dyssomnia* is characterized by the inability either to fall asleep or to stay asleep, followed by excessive daytime drowsiness. Disorders of this type include insomnia, obstructive sleep apnea, restless legs syndrome, periodic limb movement disorder, narcolepsy, and advanced and delayed sleep phase syndromes. *Parasomnias* (discussed in later chapters) are characterized by abnormalities in sleep behavior, such as night eating syndrome, night terror, sleepwalking, recurrent nightmares, sleep paralysis, bruxism (teeth grinding), and sleep talking.

INSOMNIA

Insomnia is the most common sleep disorder. You might suffer from one or any combination of insomnia's three classic types:

1. *Sleep-onset insomnia:* You have trouble falling asleep; it generally takes you more than 20 or 30 minutes to fall asleep.
2. *Early morning-awakening insomnia:* You awaken early in the morning long before you intended and are unable to get back to sleep.
3. *Sleep-maintenance insomnia:* You can't stay asleep during the night and have one or more awakenings, with trouble falling back to sleep.

OBSTRUCTIVE SLEEP APNEA

Another common sleep disorder for women, especially as we age, is *obstructive sleep apnea*. In fact, physicians often miss this diagnosis, since obstructive sleep apnea is more often associated with obese males. It occurs when airflow to the lungs is briefly blocked, most often in the throat, in repeated episodes of gasping, sometimes up to hundreds of times a night. Snoring, which does increase for aging women, is not an apnea indicator; key is the snorting sound made when gasping for air.

Symptoms of obstructive sleep apnea include excessive daytime sleepiness, waking up unrefreshed and with frequent headaches, and a dry, parched mouth. Sleep apnea factors are obesity, the use of nicotine and alcohol, use of sedating medications, hypothyroidism, sleeping on one's back, and excessive airway tissue.

If you suspect you have sleep apnea, treatments are available and include a small air pump, or CPAP, that sends you continuous positive airway pressure during sleep. Sleep apnea is serious and can affect your cardiovascular system, so treatment is important. Speak with your doctor about a possible sleep clinic referral, as a firm diagnosis is made only with an all-night monitoring.

RLS AND PLMD

Millions of women experience *restless legs syndrome* (RLS) and its companion disorder *periodic limb movement disorder*

(PLMD), which center in the lower limbs. Almost all women with RLS will have PLMD as well. With restless legs syndrome, you experience odd sensations deep within the leg muscles and knees, described as creepy-crawly, buglike sensations and/or deep itching within the leg muscles—creating forceful urges to move. RLS symptoms often get worse toward evening, preventing restful sleep. There's an urgency to get up and walk off the painful and peculiar sensations. Treatments range from hot baths, massage, and biking and stretching exercises to strict caffeine avoidance, and vitamin and mineral supplements such as iron, folic acid, calcium, and vitamin B-12 shots. Pain or tranquilizing medications are often prescribed to help blunt the brain's alerting response to the limb activity.

Periodic limb movement disorder consists of limb spasms that can occur up to hundreds of times a night. The telltale signs of PLMD are crumpled bedcovers at the foot of the bed, kicking and jerking during sleep, and excessive daytime sleepiness. Sleep-onset insomnia is common, as the limb movements continuously pull you out of stage 1 and 2 sleep. Treatment is with sedating medications.

NARCOLEPSY

Millions of women also suffer from narcolepsy, a long-term central nervous system disorder that produces an uncontrollable need to sleep during waking hours. Its three primary symptoms include (1) excessive, persistent daytime sleepiness and periodically falling asleep during normal waking hours *(sleep attacks);* (2) episodes of intense muscle weakness, collapsing in a faintlike spell *(cataplexy);* and (3) REM-phase sleep that occurs throughout the day and night *(hypnogogic hallucinations)*. These symptoms, however, are often masked by other sleep disorders, such as sleep apnea and restless legs syndrome, as excessive daytime sleepiness is blamed. Treatments include stimulant medications along with short 20-minute naps, once in the morning and again in the afternoon. (The immediate descent into REM sleep at bedtime is narcolepsy's telltale sign, diagnosed at a sleep clinic.)

Although numerous other sleep disorders have been identified, it's beyond these pages to illuminate them all. Check Resources at the back of the book for information, contact numbers, and places to start your personal research.

SEE A DOCTOR

If you are experiencing sleep troubles—whether a recent onset or chronic insomnia (persisting for more than several weeks)—the first thing to do is set up an appointment and speak with your physician. This is the best line of action and the smart thing to do.

But since much of Western, allopathic medicine seems to treat sleep difficulties as a kind of troublesome prerequisite for daily modern life, you need to be prepared and adamant about what you want: to get to the bottom of your sleep struggles. Remember that lack of sleep is not an illness but rather a symptom, like a fever.

Most likely your general practitioner has received no more than 1 or 2 hours of lecture time on this critical health issue. Until medicine catches up and primary care physicians routinely become skilled at diagnosing sleep disorders, your role as a well-informed patient is vital.

You want to rule out any medical causes for your sleep problems. Your doctor will shine here. Chemical imbalances, hormone problems, medications, and a host of medical disorders—some of which include asthma, arthritis, migraines, fibromyalgia, thyroid issues, heart disease, and diabetes—have poor sleep as a symptom. Pregnancy and menopause, though not illnesses, also affect women's sleep/wake patterns. Your doctor can help you sort through all of this.

Since sleep is often affected by medications, your doctor should know about any prescription medications and also over-the-counter remedies you take. Let her know about your supplements, diet regime, and your sleep hygiene habits (for example, whether you nap or eat late, drink caffeine or alcohol), and how and when you think your sleep problems appeared. Don't make your physician do all the detective work; you do it before you get there, and then work together.

Lack of sleep can have either a physical or a psychological cause, or some combination of the two. Once you and your physician feel confident that a physical illness and/or medication isn't the culprit, you may be referred to a sleep specialist—an M.D. with advanced training in sleep medicine—who monitors for sleep disorders such as sleep apnea, restless legs syndrome, periodic limb movement disorder, and so on, all of which are treatable to some degree.

Be open and honest about your emotional temperature and lifestyle, as well. Are you under chronic stress? Have you been a lifelong worrywart? Are you experiencing relationship struggles? Do have a history of eating disorder or addiction problems? Is there abuse in your background? Are you a workaholic? Have you suffered a major loss recently? Are you going through a divorce or experiencing some other major life stressor? Are you depressed, frustrated, or unhappy with your life?

Listen carefully to how your doctor responds to you. Does he validate your experiences and delve further, or does she minimize your experience and do all the talking? Be clear in stating what you want: You need help in regaining your optimal sleep patterns; can he help? If the only response is to take out a prescription pad and offer you sleeping pills, know that this is a temporary solution that will only mask symptoms and can cause more sleep difficulties than you have now. Discuss this concern with your doctor. Then decide what's next on your search-and-find sleep mission, knowing you'll find your way.

What if your primary care physician cannot help? Referrals are always the best, most expedient way to find a knowledgeable practitioner: specifically ask if she has skill in the area of sleep medicine or in diagnosing sleep disorders. Check the sleep foundation and health agency information in Resources, or call sleep disorder clinics in your area for referrals. Be patient but persistent, and know that you will find someone who can and will help.

CHAPTER 2

WOMEN AND SLEEP

SPECIAL ISSUES

Then sunrise kissed my Chrysalis—
And I stood up—and lived—
—EMILY DICKINSON

THERE'S NO WAY AROUND IT: YOUR HORMONES— those wonderful substances that make you a woman yet occasionally blast through your system like unrelenting tornadoes—affect your sleep. They also coordinate complex and intricate brain and body changes and fluctuate throughout your reproductive years, during pregnancy, and into and beyond menopause. Add to this biological reality work, stress, diet, marriage, children, socioeconomic pressures, and other health issues—very simply, life—and it's no wonder that delicate sleep and circadian rhythms (biological rhythms that work on an approximate 24-hour cycle and that regulate sleep, body temperature, hormone secretion, and numerous other physiological functions) are often affected. It's a wondrous, highly balanced relationship, indeed.

Although you're much more than your hormones, the cyclic rhythm of your chemical fluctuations does affect the rhythm of your slumber (as well as inflame syndromes you'll face more frequently than will a man, such as depression, anxiety, headache, and migraine). So how do the female sex hormones, estrogen and progesterone, as well as male testosterone, affect your sleep patterns?

According to sleep researchers, the brain cells involved in the sleep/wake cycle have receptors for sex hormones.

Estrogen helps women have more deep, slow-wave sleep than men, with a slower age-decline. Studies also show that estrogen enhances REM sleep (both decreasing REM onset time and increasing the duration of REM sleep). Progesterone has a sedating effect on the brain, reduces sleep onset time, and decreases nighttime awakenings. Testosterone levels also fluctuate in postmenopausal women, and some of the same symptoms experienced during estrogen loss, such as insomnia, can appear.

MENSTRUATION, PMS, AND SLEEP

Nearly every woman has experienced premenstrual syndrome, or PMS, to some degree; its symptoms occur during the early luteal phase of your cycle, two weeks prior to menstruation. (If you don't become pregnant at ovulation, both estrogen and progesterone decrease and your body sheds its uterine lining as menstrual flow.) Indications include bloating, weight gain, fluid retention, insomnia, moodiness, irritability, anxiety, headaches, acne, breast tenderness, shifts in sex drive, cramps, and cravings for carbohydrates and sweets. Studies indicate that these lowered levels of estrogen and progesterone increase nighttime awakenings and NREM, or nondream, sleep.

Recent studies also show women who suffer from PMS have less slow-wave deep sleep—stages 3 and 4—during the entire month, not just during the premenstrual weeks. The most common PMS sleep complaints include all three types of insomnia (sleep-onset, sleep-maintenance, and early morning–awakening insomnias), hypersomnia (sleeping too much), unpleasant dreams and nightmares, and morning and daytime fatigue.

If you suffer from serious mood shifts during the two weeks prior to menstruation, you may be diagnosed with premenstrual dysphoric disorder, or PMDD. While you might experience other symptoms—such as fluid retention, bloating, and cramping—with PMDD, you'll also notice mood shifts that feel like major depressions, accompanied with all the associated sleep difficulties. The symptoms disappear until the next luteal phase, when your hormones again interact to prepare your body for possible pregnancy.

~ PMS SLEEP HELP ~

For centuries women have swapped tips for dealing with their periods. Here are some suggestions to decrease PMS effects and help you sleep better during your monthly cycle.

- *Vitamins.* Increase your calcium and magnesium intake. Your body always responds favorably to calcium and magnesium, both of which help calm the central nervous system. Some studies have shown a causal link between low magnesium blood levels and PMS symptoms.
- *Fluids.* Increase your fluid intake. Water is a natural diuretic: the more you drink, the more you flush through your system. The rule of thumb is to drink approximately half your body weight, in ounces, daily. If you weigh 120 pounds, drink 60 ounces of water a day, or about 7 to 8 glasses.
- *Sodium.* Watch your sodium intake. Fluid retention is

heightened by excess sodium, so read labels carefully before you eat.

- *Diuretic herbs.* Try using a natural herbal diuretic such as dandelion, either in tablet or as a tea. Ginger, chamomile, and lemon balm teas also help with digestion and bloating.
- *Exercise.* Keep up with and even increase your exercise during your premenstrual week. Sweating helps relieve bloating, and regular exercise helps you get a deeper night's rest.
- *Bodywork.* Try some yoga and massage. The deep breathing, stretching, and meditative centering of yoga calms the nervous system and relieves abdominal and back cramping. Massage helps with lymph, fluid, and toxin drainage, and, best of all, feels wonderful. Acupuncture can also help relieve cramping.
- *Drinking.* Eliminate caffeine, carbonated drinks, and alcohol during this period. Too much caffeine and alcohol disrupt sleep patterns and exacerbate insomnia. And carbonated drinks can increase bloating and breast tenderness.
- *Eating.* Lower your carbohydrate and sugar intake. Keep away from fast foods, high-carb desserts and snacks, and chocolate (which contains not only sugar but also caffeine). As a rule, avoid high-sugar foods, which can cause a blood sugar drop that awakens you during the night.
- *B vitamins.* Take extra vitamin B6 (pyridoxine), about 100 milligrams daily. Take extra vitamin B complex during the few days before and during your period, but always check

with your physician, as taking more than 200 to 300 mg
daily of pyridoxine can be harmful.

- *Pain relief.* Take ibuprofen for the aches. This non-aspirin
pain reliever can help stave off cramps, as well as abdominal and lower back pain. Nonsteroidal anti-inflammatory
drugs, such as aspirin and ibuprofen, suppress
prostaglandins, chemicals that affect muscle tension,
which help cause menstrual cramps. Take them at bedtime
so you don't awaken during the night.

- *Fiber.* To reduce constipation, use flaxseed oil or psyllium
husks in juice or water. When you first get up, try a glass
of hot or very warm water with a little lemon and honey;
it helps flush out the system.

- *Bottle on the back.* Employ the perennial PMS trick: A hot
water bottle on the lower back does work wonders.

PREGNANCY AND SLEEP

The hormonal and bodily changes you experience with pregnancy almost inevitably mean disrupted sleep. Researchers
are beginning to collect sleep data on the three trimesters of
a normal forty-week pregnancy to determine how these
changes occur.

During the first trimester, the placenta produces high
levels of hormones, including estrogen and progesterone.
Progesterone (which has a sedating effect on the brain) levels
rise rapidly during those first twelve weeks, and most
women feel exceptionally drowsy. Many feel sufficiently
sleepy during the day that they take naps; they also tend to
sleep more hours at night.

Insomnia symptoms appear toward the end of the first trimester, as the expanding uterus starts to press on the bladder and bathroom trips become more frequent. Morning sickness, or nausea, is hormone-induced and can strike at any time, either day or night. You may suffer with backaches and tender, swollen breasts, other factors that cause sleeplessness.

Sleep improves during the second trimester as your body finally adjusts to increased hormone levels. The fetus also presses less on the bladder, necessitating fewer nighttime trips to the bathroom. But restless legs and leg cramping may appear in this part of the pregnancy, and the medication used to treat the syndrome may harm your fetus. Speak with your health-care provider about perhaps increasing iron levels to counteract painful limb sensations.

The good news is that this restless legs activity almost always subsides after pregnancy. Heartburn and gastric reflux—in which stomach acid is pushed back up from the stomach into the esophagus—can also disrupt sleep. Elevate your head slightly at night, and eat several smaller meals throughout the day.

In the third trimester, sleep deprivation and fatigue are major issues. Meanwhile, your body is still expanding, with possible frequent urination, leg cramps, heartburn, backaches, and the inability to find a comfortable sleeping position. Snoring and sleep apnea (see chapter 1) can appear; if you start to snore, have someone watch to see if you gasp for breath during the night, which lowers the oxygen not only to your brain but also to the fetus. If you live alone, you can tape-record yourself. If you indeed gasp during the night, check with your doctor about wearing a continuous airway pressure mask (CPAP) until delivery. You'll sleep better, feel less fatigued, and protect your growing baby.

As your anxiety increases over the pending delivery and new motherhood, so may instances of insomnia. It's important to do as much as you can to ease your fears. Talk to friends who have been through labor, read and gather as much information as you can, and practice some of the relaxation techniques described in this book. (A journal is particularly helpful during pregnancy and interesting to read again months and years later!) Nightmares, particularly those dealing with fears about delivery, are frequent during this last trimester, and talking through them does help.

POSTPARTUM

After delivery, both your hormones and the neurotransmitters that control mood and sleep quickly return to normal. Though the structure of your sleep changes little throughout your pregnancy and postdelivery months, sleep disruption and sleep deprivation are still big players, particularly now that you're on an extended sleep-interruption schedule for nighttime feedings. Unless you have round-the-clock help, you're going to learn firsthand all about sleep disruption once you bring your infant home. And if you already suffered with sleep disorders, you'll find them exacerbated now.

The quick drop in hormonal levels—the result of the expulsion of the hormone-secreting placenta just after birth—is thought to be a main culprit of postpartum distress, or the baby blues, about three to five or six days after birth. Most women ride out this brief period, feeling wide mood swings that usually subside and disappear after a week or so.

However, for about 10–15 percent of new mothers—particularly, those who have a history of mood disorder—these blues develop into full-blown postpartum depression, with greatly disturbed sleep. If you have a history of depression, mood disorder, or severe PMS symptoms, it's important to work with your physician and health-care providers throughout your pregnancy and during the postpartum period and beyond. You're at a much higher risk of developing serious postpartum depression, and should discuss medication and treatment with your physician.

The specific cause of postpartum depression is still unknown, though the combination of sleep deprivation, hormonal shifts, and possible labor and delivery difficulties appear to conspire to deregulate mood function.

~ PREGNANCY AND POSTPARTUM SLEEP HELP ~

Use all the healthy lifestyle choices, sleep strategies, and relaxation techniques you've ever learned during and after your pregnancy. You'll need them. Here are a few to make special note of.

- *Sleep on your left side.* The National Sleep Foundation recommends sleeping on your left side during pregnancy to allow the best blood flow to the uterus and kidneys. Most women find putting a pillow between their legs— special pregnancy pillows are available—helps reduce backaches, which can wake you up.
- *Take naps.* Make use of naps to offset your sleep

fragmentation, both during pregnancy and postpartum. The advice "Sleep when your baby sleeps" holds true; and if you can bring in someone to help during your naptime, all the better. Don't feel guilty about your sleep needs. Take advantage of any social and family support you can.

- *Eat well.* Obviously, make sure you're eating good, nutritious food that has a positive effect on your quality of sleep. Avoid high-sugar and spicy foods, particularly late in the evening, drink plenty of water up until dinner, and eat smaller meals more often.

- *Exercise.* Keep on a regular exercise routine to improve circulation and help you sleep deeply. Don't push too hard, and make sure you warm up and cool down, and use good breathing techniques.

- *Avoid stimulants.* Avoid caffeine, nicotine, and alcohol. These can harm your fetus and nursing baby, as well as disrupt your sleep. If you absolutely must have some kind of caffeinated drink, ask your doctor or health-care provider how much caffeine you can safely consume.

- *Explore bodywork and movement.* With the enormous changes your body has undergone, massage and acupuncture can help restore balance to your system. Movement class, dance, and yoga—sometimes geared for pregnancy or postpregnancy needs—also smoothes out major body transformation and transition.

- *Get your sleep.* Practice good sleep habits, and make consistent use of relaxation routines. These are important healthy lifestyle choices, particularly during pregnancy and early motherhood. Make sleep a priority, and learn to share nighttime duties with a partner, if possible (you can breast-pump milk for night feedings).

- *Ask for help.* If serious sleep deprivation persists, consider asking someone to come in one night a week or bi-monthly (perhaps different friends and/or relatives) so you can get at least several good, solid sleep nights each month.

PERIMENOPAUSE, MENOPAUSE, AND SLEEP

As your body did with the onset of your menstruation, it will decide when you experience menopause, technically the cessation of menstrual periods for a full year. Perimenopause, or the years leading up to the menopausal marker, can begin anywhere from four to ten years earlier than your last menstrual cycle. During these years, you'll notice physical changes as your ovaries start to decrease production of estrogen and progesterone.

The most common menopausal symptom—hot flashes (along with night sweats)—occurs for about 80 percent of the 50 million women moving through menopause and is the one symptom most associated with insomnia. Studies clearly show that perimenopausal and menopausal women have a much higher incidence of sleep disturbance and insomnia than do premenopausal women. These sleep disruptions are often associated with hot flashes' quick rise in body temperature (which can occur up to hundreds nightly), since a lowered body temperature promotes sleep.

When estrogen (along with progesterone) is replaced through traditional hormone replacement therapy (HRT) or through more natural plant extracts, menopausal symptoms often decrease. Estrogen replacement is particularly effective for hot flashes and insomnia. Along with many health benefits—such as protection against heart disease, stroke, osteoporosis, and hypertension—estrogen replacement has also been shown to significantly improve sleep.

However, HRT is not recommended for women who have a personal or family history of breast cancer, uterine cancer, blood clots, and/or liver disease. Many other women choose to forgo estrogen replacement because of the documented increase in risk for breast cancer. Still, there are menopausal hormone supplements and treatments available that will help with sleep, some traditional, some alternative; most notably, Chinese herbs and acupuncture.

~ PERIMENOPAUSE AND MENOPAUSE ~
SLEEP HELP

- *Herbals.* Herbs like fennel, dong quai, red clover, and black cohosh are phytoestrogens and can help reduce hot flashes, insomnia, and other symptoms. Health food stores often carry the herbs in preformulated supplements, or you can take them through teas. Always check with your physician before taking any herbal supplement; women who are on HRT are cautioned against using phytoestrogens.

- *Soy.* Increase your soy protein intake. Research shows that an increase of soy to the diet lessens the frequency and intensity of hot flashes and thus helps reduce nighttime awakenings.

- *Vitamins.* Many gynecologists suggest taking an extra 200 mg of time-released vitamin B6 (pyridoxine) to reduce the side effects of hormone replacement therapy. Extra vitamin E, as well as extra calcium and magnesium, may also help with symptoms. Again, make sure you consult with your physician first.

- *Nightclothes.* If you suffer from hot flashes, breathable cotton pajamas and sheets are better than synthetic fabrics. Use loose, light bed clothing, and keep an extra pair of pajamas or a nightshirt by the bed so you can quickly change clothes after a nighttime drenching.

- *Good sleep hygiene.* Excellent sleep hygiene accentuates the positive during these sometimes negative sleep years: eat properly; exercise regularly; use relaxation techniques to reduce stress and discomfort; go to bed and rise at the same time; avoid late-night eating and stimulants, such as caffeine, nicotine, and sugar, as well as alcohol.

- *Bodywork.* Acupuncture and regular massage help many women sleep better throughout midlife hormonal shifts. Shiatsu massage and reflexology are two good choices. Daily yoga and stretching exercise, morning and evening, help relieve tension and calm the nervous system.

SENIOR WOMEN AND SLEEP

Older women often unwittingly alter their circadian rhythms once they hit retirement age or reduce their daily schedules. The frequency and length of naps increases at age sixty-five and older, and the normal biological rhythms shift, with shortened circadian rhythms appearing. This shift is called Advanced Phase Disorder and means sleepiness appears around 8 P.M. rather than II P.M. Of course, this also means that the early morning waking hour shifts forward, and suddenly you find yourself waking up at 4 A.M. instead of 7. It's a frustration for many women. What to do?

Exposure to bright light will help reset your biological clock. Early morning walks are excellent, as are those in the late afternoon, right before dusk. Follow the sun as much as possible. Reduce or eliminate naps. Regular evening hot baths will help induce sleep as well, but be sure to check with your doctor if you have high blood pressure, a heart condition, or if you're prone to dizziness. Both you and your physician should go over your medications, supplements, and over-the-counter pills, all of which can impact the quality of your sleep.

Once in bed, practice relaxation exercises and deep breathing. If you awaken throughout the night in order to go to the bathroom (overactive bladder is a problem in this age group), check to make sure you really need to go or if it's just become habit. If you do think you have an overactive bladder, ask your doctor for possible medication. And if you often wake up too early in the morning, don't lie in bed and fill your mind with worry; get up and start your day out in the sunlight. Work with your health-care professional to set up a circadian rhythm shift for several weeks: early morning and dusk walks, no afternoon naps, a hot bath at the earlier sleepy time, and a later bedtime. Eventually, your rhythm will shift over.

SLEEP AND ADRENAL HEALTH

Many women don't consider the impact of adrenal health on sleep. The adrenal glands, located above the kidneys, generate the powerful stress hormone cortisol, whose natural arc—elevated in the morning, lower in the evening—helps provide daytime energy and nighttime sleep. However, insomnia and sleeplessness occur if stress is causing your adrenal glands to lock into overdrive, producing too much cortisol throughout the day and evening. In longer lasting stages, this is termed "adrenal exhaustion."

Hormonal imbalance is one result of adrenal exhaustion, leading to hot flashes, night sweats, mood swings, and insomnia. If you suspect adrenal overload, check with your physician to see if you can take a saliva test to check your sex hormones and cortisol levels; this will give both of you an idea of how to proceed in rebuilding your adrenal function. In the meantime, taking a good multivitamin and mineral tablet along with extra vitamin C and B complex can help.

DEPRESSION AND MOOD DISORDER

Disturbed sleep—either insomnia and hyposomnia (too much sleep)—is the classic hallmark of depression. And whereas most everyone experiences a period of low mood, or the blues, at some point in life, there's a clear distinction between the occasional depression and a major depressive disorder, which is a type of mood disorder. Think of the difference as a transient bout with headache versus chronic, unremitting migraine.

Clinical depression is a serious, debilitating illness. Fortunately, it is also treatable. It can occur in anyone, though twice as many women than men suffer from it—approximately 12 million American women yearly. Depression's key symptom is a marked shift in mood that is both severe and persistent. You might notice a sense of lethargy, or you no longer take pleasure in everyday events and friends. You may have trouble concentrating and feel increasingly anxious. For a diagnosis of clinical depression, these symptoms generally must remain unabated for two weeks.

If you suspect you may have a major depressive disorder, it's crucial you contact a qualified physician or health-care provider and seek treatment. Today, there is no need to suffer through such an illness alone. Treatments include antidepressant medication with either a serotonin reuptake inhibitor (SSRI) such as Prozac or a tricyclic, such as Elavil, along with psychotherapy and many alternative health possibilities (see Resources). Once the depression lifts, your sleep will regain its regularity.

SEASONAL AFFECTIVE DISORDER

During the winter months, seasonal affective disorder (SAD) appears in about 15 million people, once again in more women than men. It's a depressive syndrome that patterns itself with seasonal light cycles. When light diminishes in winter months, the syndrome increases. SAD symptoms are like those of depression but with several major differences: SAD sufferers have an increased need for an almost hibernating sleep—sometimes up to 9 or 10 hours, though they find that it rarely refreshes them; their carbohydrate cravings substantially increase, particularly during the early and late evening; and they feel the need for long afternoon naps.

Phototherapy, or light therapy (see chapter 5), is the treatment of choice, often with full-spectrum, indoor bright lights timed in the early morning hours for 20 minutes at a time. The bright light tricks the brain into thinking it is summer. If sunlight is available, early morning and sunset walks, without sunglasses, are also advised.

Now that you're armed with some basic knowledge about how your sleeping brain works—and how the sleeping process can become subverted—the following sixty suggestions will help you gain the rest and deep sleep you desire.

4

CHAPTER 3

CREATING THE RIGHT ENVIRONMENT

GET A NEW MATTRESS

May your bed sprout onions.
—YIDDISH CURSE

A NICE, NEW, BEAUTIFUL MATTRESS WILL DO more for your sleep than you might think. Today, we have the fallacious idea that mattresses are like refrigerators: buy one every thirty years! That's fine if your mattress holds up solid for that long, but more than likely it won't. I know people who will spend hundreds of dollars on a pair of shoes and yet complain they can feel the springs in their mattresses. Forget it. Be honest, and if you need to get a new mattress—go out and get one.

You'll find no shortage of choice when purchasing your mattress. It's a virtual supermarket out there—soft, firm, super-support, temperature-controlled—everyone gets a choice, and if you have sleep difficulties, your mattress choice is critical. Many people like the fluidness of waterbeds; others love sleeping on the floor, Japanese style, which gives excellent back support. Try experimenting before making your next bedding choice and investment.

If you do choose a traditional spring-coil mattress, look for a model at least seven inches thick, with a minimum of 300 coils for full-size, 375 for a queen, and 450 coils for a king. Flip and rotate your mattress two to four times yearly, and be sure to do at least a thorough annual or bi-annual vacuuming and airing. This is important. You want to avoid anything to do with dust and dust mites. Always use a mattress pad; the thick and hypo-allergenic ones are best.

And every woman knows that what goes on top of the bed is almost as important as the mattress underneath. I've always believed a bed is a kind of life microcosm, a personal fiefdom, so who wants a boring bed? Splurge. No need to be prosaic when there's so much plumage around. Sumptuous down comforters, goose feather pillows, silk or satin sheets, cashmere blankets all make sleep time more desirous.

It only makes sense to spend some money investing in what you'll spend one-third of your life on and in. And if you take good care of your bedding, particularly the more expensive, delicate pieces, using soft detergents and removing them from the dryer while still slightly damp, they can last decades.

Of course, there's no proof you will sleep one minute longer or better on an expensive, well-crafted mattress, piled with down comforters and covered with 450-count vermilion Egyptian cotton sheets, than on plain sturdy Army whites, but I say leave that proof for someone with nothing else to do.

USE YOUR BED ONLY FOR SLEEP

'Tis very warm weather when one is in bed.
—JONATHAN SWIFT

THE CONCEPT OF BED ADDICTION COMES AS A surprise to many; most people who struggle with sleep rarely realize how much time they actually spend on and around or thinking about their beds. Insomniacs have a love/hate relationship with beds, and it seems to come out at night, full force.

A sleep disorder specialist once asked how much time I spend on my bed while not sleeping. I had never considered the question before. Of course, I like to watch TV for a couple of hours lounging on the bed, who doesn't? Yes, I do talk on the phone, like to eat, love to read (is there a better place to read a book?). I suddenly got the picture, and it wasn't pretty.

The doctor's orders: Get out of bed with a set alarm, immediately make the bed, and *do not go near the bed again until you're ready to sleep.* "No way," I howled. "That's impossible!" The doctor smiled and said, "It sounds like I'm asking you to give up heroin." "Well, you are!" He suggested if I had that strong of a reaction to the mere possibility of giving up bed-lounging, I should consider whether my relationship with my bed might just be a little off. The next day, I did what he suggested, and within a few weeks I was sleeping much better.

In sleep medicine it's called "bed restriction." The routine is this: Set your alarm the night before. When it goes off in the morning, get out of bed. Immediately make your bed, and *do not go near your bed again for any reason* until you are ready to sleep. Do nothing else on your bed. Period. Do not even perch on the bedside to tie your shoes; you can do that somewhere else! This one rather simple routine will help your mind and body reassociate bed with uniform sleep—a crucial lesson in the battle for nighttime slumber.

Go through your bedroom, and you might be surprised to see how much you've set up your life around your bed. Television, telephone, books, magazines, remote controls, lamps, work papers, laptops, CD players, cell phones—why are they all within reach of your bed? If you sense this is a snapshot of your bedroom, clear things out and rearrange the furniture, literally and figuratively.

It doesn't matter if your bed addiction is stronger or weaker than anyone else's. If you spend any time on or around or thinking about your bed other than during the physical act of sleeping in it, your bed-and-sleep relationship is polluted with extraneous bed activities. No doubt it's an emotional issue, but you should take crisp physical remedial action.

So forget thinking about your bed, lying on your bed, taking comfort and succor from your bed, except while you're asleep, at least for the time being. Only after you become a long-time good, deep sleeper can you jump back onto your emotive raft. But by that time, you won't even give it a second thought.

PURIFY YOUR AIR

Insomnia is when both sides of
the pillow feel hot.
—ANNA AKHMATOVA

I F YOU LIVE IN THE COUNTRY, AWAY FROM CARS,
smog, CO_2, and pollution in general, congratulations.
This suggestion is not for you. But if you're like most of
us, stuck deep inside a city or a suburb, pollution and bad air
are things you must learn to live with.

If you live in any situation where you feel you're being
pummeled by air pollution or carbon monoxide—from cars,
old heaters (particularly check for these if you live in an old
apartment), garages—take action quickly. Carbon monoxide
poisoning is deadly serious (you can't smell it in the air), and
you don't have to be poisoned to death to have extremely
disturbed sleep from higher levels of gas in your home's air.

Plants are nature's carbon monoxide cleaners and natural
air purifiers. In my early adult years, I'm sure plants saved my
life more than once in the variety of exotic places I resided.
Have as many plants as you think you can take care of, but
also remember that past a certain point they compete with
you for oxygen. So don't go overboard.

Dust, musty drapes, bedding, carpets are all containers for
dirt and dust—and all contribute to bedroom air pollution.
It's common to let beds get surrounded with books and

magazines and paraphernalia; move the clutter around and dust it off. So if you're not by nature a hausfrau, at least make sure your sleeping area is continuously clean, or pay someone to come in and do it for you regularly.

Many people swear by the new, silent air purifiers currently on the market. They're generally expensive, but if you have allergies, are especially sensitive to airborne pollutants, or if you're in a situation where—despite your best efforts—your bedroom air will remain less than clean, purchase one. It's your health and sleep, after all.

Check the temperature in your bedroom, too. Middle-of-the-road air temperature is best, neither too hot nor too cold. A temperature between 68 and 77 degrees is best. Recall that a fall in body temperature is what helps you go to sleep and stay asleep, so you don't want a warm, stuffy room heating you up. If one partner seems to have descended from penguins and the other from Sahara Bedouins, keep the room cool and give the cold partner a blanket.

BAN THE CLOCK

Fatigue is the best pillow.
—BENJAMIN FRANKLIN

I OFTEN WONDER WHY TIME IS SO OF THE ESSENCE in bedrooms—or rather knowing what time it is. Is there any other room in the house that has so many timepieces? Your bathroom? The garage?

Modern bedroom time invader number one: new digital clocks that glow each passing minute in flashy, unpleasant red or green. There's one on your VCR; turn your head and there it glows on your AM/FM radio clock. You no doubt have a bedside alarm; perhaps there's also a desk clock; and then there's your watch on your dresser table. Add five more. If you have a computer that remains on all night, add an additional timepiece.

So in one bedroom, there are six timepieces that all scream the same thing all night long: It's 2 A.M. and you're not asleep. I'm a firm believer that bedrooms should be time-free environments. Today, with so many seemingly conflicting family schedules, this may seem almost impossible. However, if your bedroom can't be completely time-free, it should at least be less time-strident.

Time really should be of little importance to you at night. I know this seems unfair to insomniacs who latch much of their critical thinking and mental obsessions to clocks and time, but that's exactly why banning clocks—and particularly glow-in-the-dark bedroom clocks—is such a good idea.

Don't sabotage your sleep any more than you have to. If you need to awaken on time, set an alarm clock and turn it around on the bed table; or better yet, put it inside a drawer or under the bed or bedroom chair—best, across the room, someplace where you can't just flip it around to satisfy your curiosity every half-hour.

Everyone wakes up during the night—in actuality after every REM period—so you awaken briefly about four to five times a night. Most people just shift sleep positions and go back to sleep, not remembering waking up. But for people who have trouble sleeping, no such luck. There's that bright clock to tell you exactly what time it is and how little you have left before the alarm does go off.

Before I learned this trick, I woke up at exactly 3 A.M. every morning for two years. Doctors were suspicious, but it's true. How did I know? I looked at the glowing red digital wonder across from my bed. See! It's 3 A.M. Like Pavlov's dog, I conditioned myself to wake up at that exact time to see that exact number on the clock. It's truly a joy never to have to see those red numbers say 3 A.M. ever again. One, because the clock is no longer there; two, usually at that time, I'm now fast asleep.

So do yourself a favor, declare your bedroom a time-free zone. At the very least, you'll fall back to sleep a lot more easily if you don't know if it's 2 A.M., 2:04 A.M., or 2:05 A.M. Just know when it's dark, you should be asleep.

TURN OFF THE ELECTRICITY

❧

Computers are useless. They can only
give you answers.
—PABLO PICASSO

WE'VE ALL HEARD THE ADAGE IF A BUTTERFLY flaps its wings in Hong Kong, there's a hurricane in Manhattan. Today, quantum physics verifies this fact, telling us the world is vitalized by an unending spiral of energy intermingled and never lost. For better sleep, be conscious of the electromagnetic forces surrounding you, the energy interchange that occurs whether you see and feel it or not.

Think of your bedroom and how much energy from electronic equipment is jamming up your air. You think you can't feel it and it has no effect on you, but Western physics and ancient Asian philosophies and medicine say otherwise. Ideally, you'll have as few pieces of electronic equipment in your bedroom as possible. Zero would be the best number. Yet, today, this seems highly impractical. So compromise.

If you're a good consumer, you'll have a television, radio, stereo, VCR or DVD player, a portable phone or two, a portable tape player by your bed for early morning jogging, a clock radio, an answering machine . . . If you have a work station in part of your bedroom there's probably a computer, fax, printer, copy machine, scanner—and this is likely all in a relatively small space.

Again, be aware that all these units—particularly the television and computer—give off high levels of electromagnetic energy, even long after they've been shut off. Studies show prolonged exposure to electromagnetic energy fields can cause immune-related illnesses, let alone disturb sleep.

Tally up and see how many pieces of electronic equipment you have in your bedroom, and then clear out as many as you can. If you must have a television in your bedroom, put it in an entertainment center or cupboard where you can shut the doors; or if it must be free-standing, place a cloth or piece of fabric over the screen at night.

Plants also help absorb some of this electrical pollution: the rule of thumb is one big plant per item of electronic equipment. Palms, peace lilies, and spider plants are said to absorb the most electrical charges.

If you cannot remove your computer, fax, printer, and other work-related electronics, at the very least diligently turn off the machines at night, turn the computer screen around, and cover it with a plastic cover. Make sure all electronic pieces—and that includes clock radios and portable phones—are at least four feet from where you rest your head while asleep.

I do have a computer in my bedroom and at first inadvertently placed the screen a couple of feet from the head of my bed. Turning the screen around, moving it four feet away, covering the screen at night, and consistently turning it off absolutely did improve the quality of my sleep. Madison Avenue will never tell you about electromagnetic fields when they try to sell you the latest entertainment gadget, which inevitably gets placed in the bedroom; buyer and sleeper beware.

STOP WATCHING
THE LATE-NIGHT NEWS

If you wish to drown, do not torture
yourself with shallow water.

—BULGARIAN POEM

I S THERE ANY REASON YOU CAN THINK OF TO
watch the news late at night, right before you go to
sleep? Even if it were good news, which it is not, it
would still stir up your mind before rest. In the twenty-first
century, we have the strange luxury of hearing about stab-
bings, murder, rape, abusive parents, mayhem, war, scandal,
violent crime—all dished up in tabloidish form—parading
as "news" at 11 P.M. Good grief, it's time to stop.

The day I made the decision to stop watching the late-
evening news at bedtime, I immediately not only slept better
but also felt better, cleaner, lighter, more refreshed. Sure, I
might not know about every murder that takes place in my
city nor be hip to the latest political sound bite. But I figure
if it's worth knowing, it's worth waiting to know about in
the morning.

The way I see it, the more the world is viewed through
the media, the more it appears as careening out of control.
We're stunned into forgetting that there have always been
murderers, rapists, sociopaths galore, and every generation
must have thought theirs the most monumental and crazed.

Bad news and stress are nothing new. Yet since global angst is now available at every moment, a survival, stressed, satiated mind-set bangs away, so opposed to gentle sleep.

If you really want to go all the way, and think you can handle it, try a "news fast." This is where you don't watch TV news, read the newspaper, check the Internet news sites, listen to the radio, or ask your friends to fill you in on the day's happenings. Rather, just revel in the fact that the world is turning just fine, without you knowing about every single thing that's happening just this minute. Surprisingly, news junkies often find this task not too difficult to carry out. And just as when you return from a food fast and your taste buds are more perceptive and healthy, so, too, will you be more aware of news dross.

Make a unilateral decision to stop watching the late-night news at bedtime, and you'll see how much better you sleep and how much better you feel in general. This is an easy one to give up, and the results are pleasantly surprising.

CREATE A BEDTIME RITUAL

*Make your own beautiful footprints
in the snow.*
— BARBARA KIMBALL

DON'T BE SURPRISED IF YOU GET A BLANK stare in response to the question, What's your bedtime ritual? To many, a bedtime ritual might be hopping into bed and turning out the lights. That would be fine if all you did all day was loll around the garden, living an unruffled life. Even then, though, you'd be missing out on a joyous part of the day.

Rituals are a kind of primeval exercise that promote feelings of safety, relaxation, joy, connectedness. They help people let down their guard. Think of how many millions of rituals exist in the world today—from throughout history—and how much they resist elimination. For sleep, these ritual cues are very important. They not only help you switch gears by slowly relaxing you and removing that daytime armor, but they're also a creative and pleasing part of the day.

I bet you can remember your favorite childhood bedtime ritual. Likely it went something like this: Put on your pajamas, brush your teeth, climb in bed, listen to a bedtime story, say good night to each of your stuffed friends, prayer time, a hug and kiss good night, your parent saying, "See you later, alligator," "After a while, crocodile." Then you take out your flashlight and read and/or tell jokes and giggle with your siblings, until you hear, "Alright, you two, knock it off." Then it's really time to go to sleep.

How many times did you enact the ritual? Who knows, and yet it created safe and relaxing wind-down time to prepare you for sleep. These are great sleep habits.

Why then, as adults, do people think they can skip a prolonged bedtime ritual? Again, if you have problems sleeping, bedtime wind-down routines are vital. Working until 11 P.M. and turning off your computer isn't going to cut it as a ritual. You need at least an hour, better two, to start turning off your mind, letting go of the day, and switching gears to dark, night, rest, and sleep.

Here's where your private thumbprint comes in. Your rituals can be as elaborate or as simple as you want. Reading is probably a top candidate, along with stretching and deep breathing. Lots of people I know answer e-mails and return phone calls to friends, but, personally, I'd find that too stimulating. Playing with your children, working on a novel, needlework, journal writing are all wonderful wind-down routines.

Working late to meet journalistic deadlines is sometimes tough, but I try to stop at least two hours before sleep. I take a short walk, have a hot bath, do some yoga, paint in my studio, write in my journal, daydream a bit, and the last thing I do is write my to-do list for the next day. I hop in bed, read, listen to music, and then, the sound of silence. It sounds dry in sentence form, but it's actually a luscious part of the day.

There are endless ways to create your own bedtime ritual. Create one, stamp it yours, and regularize it. Most of all, enjoy it.

BRING IN CANDLES

❧

It is better to light a candle
than curse the darkness.
—CHINESE PROVERB

ANDLELIGHT IS PROBABLY ONE OF THE MOST
soothing and sensual nighttime rituals you'll come
across.

It was the world's only light until Edison invented fluo-
rescent light bulbs, a kind of modern light, incidentally, that
the brain does not even register as light waves. It makes sense,
then, that the nighttime part of our evolved brain is highly
susceptible to candlelight during darkness, particularly when
preparing for sleep.

Scented candles have lovely aromas—and you can buy
just about any earthly scent from myrrh to Moroccan jasmine—but the point here is focusing on soft light. Turn off
the light bulbs in your room, lie or sit down either on the
floor or in bed just before nodding off, and stare into the
soft, natural, flickering light. Let your eyes and mind rest on
the light, drinking it in.

Zen masters tell you focusing on a single object frees the
mind; it has a double effect here, as soft light warms the eyes
and relaxes the spirit. Let your mind wander for 5 minutes,
and then take another 5 minutes and try to meditate, letting
go of all thought. Just make sure you blow out that candle

before you fall asleep, and if there's any question you may drift off with the candle still lit, stay out of bed during the short meditation.

A few things to remember when purchasing candles: Inexpensive candles are fine, but if you plan on consistently using one candle, splurge and spend the extra money. You'll get not only a cleaner burning candle (check to make sure wicks are lead-free, you don't want smokestacks) but also a longer burning candle (an average $15 candle burns approximately 20 hours, and a $40 candle about 50 hours). Also, if you refrigerate candles for a few hours, they'll burn more evenly and slowly.

With so many candle choices today, your pick is your fancy. Look for exotic fragrances such as blackcurrant, vanilla, Moroccan orange, sweet jasmine, golden bamboo, citrus, caramel, tangerine, tonka beans, and brown sugar (some of my favorites). You can always play it safe with scents like lavender, ylang-ylang, Bulgarian rose, sandalwood, or gardenia.

Keep candles strewn throughout your bedroom; lighting various fragrances in different spots on different days is a lovely way to end the night. Perhaps you'll want to say a prayer as you light a candle or whisper a blessing as you blow out the light. Feel lucky someone created something as beautiful as a candle.

DISCOVER FENG SHUI

*We shape our buildings;
thereafter they shape us.*
—WINSTON CHURCHILL

FENG SHUI IS A COMPLEX, 3,000-YEAR-OLD Chinese philosophy based on the art of placement, harmony, balance, and the fundamental principle that cosmic energy *(chi)* unites all universal matter. In Feng Shui's system, nothing happens without direct consequence to something else; free-flowing *chi* that circulates smoothly has positive influence on everything in its path. Stagnant *chi* or *chi* that moves too rapidly has a negative effect on your well-being. Harnessing good *chi* and directing its flow is in large part Feng Shui's goal.

And like the Western approach to yoga—another complex, centuries-old system—people take from Feng Shui what works best for their lives. You might find some things in Feng Shui superstitious and others good intuitive sense: simply use what feels right for you.

In this system, your bedroom is the most important room in your home, as this is where you sleep and renew your body. It's the one space you inhabit that's completely yours, the outside world kept at bay. It should be tranquil, peaceful, and inspire proper rest, privacy, and your true personality. Here are some Feng Shui bedroom and sleep principles:

- Bed placement is key. Most important, never have the foot of your bed in direct alignment with the door. This is known as the "death" or "coffin" position and suggests your *chi* will flow straight out of the room while sleeping. (I have heard many people say this one switch works wonders.)

- From the bed's headboard position you should have full view of both the windows and the door. Try to place the bed against a solid wall, making sure headboards are tightly fastened to the frames. Never place a bed directly under a low-slanting ceiling, a window, or under exposed beams, as this is thought to dilute *chi* by half.

- Place your bed so your head points north to ensure your body's axis is parallel to the Earth's and is in direct line to receive the magnetic energy swinging through the Earth at the North Pole. The north–south axis is said to have a quiet, more peaceful energy and helps promote restful sleep. Charles Dickens apparently knew this, as he purportedly always traveled with a compass and adamantly turned all his beds north–south.

- Your bed is the one piece of furniture in your home that pulls the most energy from you—you spend one-third of your life on it—so Feng Shui masters suggest changing your bed mattress every time a new life cycle starts, approximately every seven to nine years, and especially if you bring a new partner into your bed. Also, whenever you move, try to buy a new mattress.

- A major Feng Shui rule: Do not leave beds unmade. This stagnates and erodes *chi* as well as looks un-wonderful. It's the very first thing I do in the morning, and if nothing else, do it respectfully for yourself.
- Feng Shui principles suggest sparing use of mirrors in the bedroom: one mirror is the maximum, something unusual for Westerners. Don't have mirrors face the bed, as they reflect and increase *chi* and disturb sleep. *Chi* escapes from windows, so you want to cover them at night. Try to keep the sharp edges of bedroom furniture from pointing toward the sleeper.
- Clutter and electronic equipment stagnate and erode *chi*-flow: cover your television and computer screens with plastic covers or draped cloths, and hang a crystal ball just above your bedroom's clutter spot. Also, keep the underside of your bed clear—don't store things under your bed. Use a closet.

If you find your interest piqued by this information, there are numerous books and Feng Shui experts to help you increase your "bedroom *chi*." NOTE: Feng Shui bed placement is complex, with multiple compass directions and quadrants to consider. I advise reading a complete chapter on the subject.

LISTEN TO LULLABIES AT BEDTIME

There's a lullaby made to calm the ruler
of sharper things.
−JOY HARPO

S OUND IS ONE OF YOUR MOST SOOTHING SENSES, and soothing, soft music is sound to put you to slumber. Remember lullabies? You can have your own adult form each night by starting a routine of listening to supple sounds just before sleep.

Isn't there something about bedtime and singing, music and lulling sound that feels like a brain balm, a fused childhood melody? Perhaps parents just want to hear the sound of their own voices singing, but for whatever reason, children crave this soft, singing sound, and I think it never goes away. Mine sits undulled in the rose quartz of my kid heart.

If you have a tape deck or CD player by your bed, once you crawl under the covers, flip something in and lie back, relax and let your mind float. Sacred choral music is perfect for this: Mozart, Handel, any rich and gorgeous work will do. *A capella* voices are luminescent and most closely resemble real lullabies. Of course, anything in Italian and by Boccelli is on the list. Stringed classical music is highly meditative: violins, cello, flutes, oboe, even soft drums are lulling and shushing.

There are records of beautiful rainforest sounds, sounds from the oceans and underwaters, African animal night-chanting, and private nature mysticisms, such as storm clouds and the wind. Many instrumentals now have mothers' heartbeats and cooing doves embedded in them. It's called "white noise" and is suggested by many sleep specialists.

What's important is no oompah or revelry music, nothing stimulating or pulsating, so save the hip-hop to get you going in the morning. Think celestial, classical, sacred, soft, lulling—and then have them ready by your bed at night, to just pick up and put on the earphones.

Building your own lullaby library has never been easier: you can buy songs from every imaginable place on the planet, all which had mothers and fathers who sung their children to sleep. Celtic, Scottish, Welsh, Manx lullabies are wondrous; in the Celtic cultures the suantrai (sleep music) was considered one of music's three main categories. African, Brazilian, Javanese, Yiddish, bamboo flute lullabies from Japan—I even have a recording from Greenland. The same love and mythic charm runs through them all.

It's the each and every wish of a lullaby (in Gaelic): *mi gysgl di 'maban* (you'll sleep my baby) *a 'r bore a ddaw* (and the morning will come).

~ COUNT SHEEP ~

*I really can't be expected to drop everything and
start counting sheep at my age. I hate sheep.*
—DOROTHY PARKER

I wonder if anyone really does count those fuzzy little
lambs jumping over fences? Wherever and however this
quirky mind trick got started, it is, in actuality, a self-
patterning, repetitive, hypnotic suggestion that does work.

Counting sheep—or some imaginative version of
sheep—combines two potent self-hypnosis techniques:
visualizing a peaceful, bucolic scene and the mantra-ish
repetition of mathematics and numbers. Counting sheep
is one ancient trick probably everyone who's been unable
to get to sleep has used at one time or another.

Counting sheep, by the way, is not the same thing as
visualization, where there is more of an active plotline and,
often times, cast members. Here, it's the drone and repeti-
tiveness of the images, not the dazzle, that counts.

My version of counting sheep: The minute my head
hits the pillow, my mind automatically starts searching for
something both pleasing and repetitive; sometimes I shift
the poems I write and hoard in licorice-colored notebooks;
sometimes I clear clothes out of my jammed closet. Other
times I list books I want to read, replant my back garden,
anything that keeps my mind moving through a scene, and
at some arbitrary point, my mind gets satisfied and floats
onto something else. If all else fails, I start reciting favorite
childhood poems, usually from *Alice in Wonderland*.

Is this boring? Of course. That's the point of counting sheep: boredom, and eventually sleep.

One girlfriend tells me she makes up names for her unborn children. My more plodding friends go over taxes, shift furniture, redo grocery lists. A male friend says he plays the world's most famous golf courses, hole by hole, until he's under. Orthodox or unorthodox, who cares? It keeps your mind off transient worries and onto things with no emotional pull.

However you do it, this sheep-counting technique works. At least on good nights. Experiment and let your mind go. Sooner or later you'll land on something your mind enjoys repeating again and again. Just keep it soft and quiet and positive. If all else fails, you can start naming the sheep.

SET REGULAR WAKE-UP CALLS

*There is nobody who totally lacks
the courage to change.*

−ROLLO MAY

YOU PROBABLY KNOW THIS TYPE OF SLEEP braggart: "Me, never had a problem sleeping. Sleep like a log. Always have. Couldn't sleep past 6 A.M. if I tried." Insomniacs and troubled sleepers find this concept hard to fathom. But what lies squarely at the heart of this scenario is a consistent pattern of regular, daily established wake time that the body and brain—and your circadian rhythm—learned through good sleep habits.

It's called "good sleep hygiene," and every sleep disorder specialist will tell you up front, if you have problems sleeping, set a regular wake-up time and stick to it, no operatic excuses. Set an alarm, three if you have to, and when it goes off, get out of bed. Period. It's one of the standard hallmarks of sleep therapy, and if you're serious about getting to a state like the sleep braggart mentioned, there's really no way around it.

The reason is this: Your body temperature begins its rise when you wake and become active, and if you delay this for several hours, your body temperature drop in the evening drops that much later. You want to establish a consistent rise-and-fall body temperature rhythm that helps you sleep both more deeply and more refreshed.

If you have a varied schedule—particularly if you work from home and have the option of waking up to cold alarms or cooing birds—organize and settle this issue now. (I've yet to hear anyone experience what many of us might fantasize: a soft, angelic voice whispering at the same time each morning: "Time to wake up.") It's simple: If the birds don't wake you up at the same time each morning, let the alarm.

Here's the easy part: Figure out how much sleep you need and set your alarm accordingly. Here's the nonnegotiable: Get into bed at the proper time, and no matter what your sleep was like—even if you got only 1 hour—when the alarm goes off, bedtime is over. Get up out of bed. This might seem harsh and unforgiving—not to say exceptionally difficult at first. But without question, this regular-rising rhythm will dramatically improve your sleep.

Do yourself a favor: Do the math and set your alarm and rise out of bed at the same time for six months. If the sleep doctors are correct, it'll be like the wings on an airplane to better, more restful sleep.

CHAPTER 4

DE-STRESSING
THE MIND

BEFRIEND TIME

*You thought growing older would be
more of the same . . . tonight will not be
the equal of last night, even in sleep.*
—HAYDEN CARRUTH

LAST WEEK I DROVE PAST A BILLBOARD ADVERTIS-
ing a new handheld computer: "We make instantaneous faster!" The minute I read that sentence I felt
exhausted. I knew it wasn't some sort of sardonic joke; they
meant exactly what they said. The lure was in the insanity.

This overachieving state of affairs, with its focus on
"faster," "more," "higher," "now," "first," portrays the person
who saunters through time as an undesirable underachiever.
There is a balance—learning to understand and value time
for what it is and what it can and cannot do for you—but if
you want to learn to sleep, deeply and soundly, start leaning
toward the slower-paced side of that equation. Concentrate
on letting time flow smoothly rather than gush and stop and
spurt along.

After all, time has never even been proven, either by
physicists or philosophers, to run in a straight linear line, moving from left to right, past to present to future. Clock-time
is an invention of man—and it wasn't until the twelfth century that Benedictine monks created clocks for their daily
offices. To become a slave to an invention, even something as

seductive as time, only bespeaks another addiction. For the insomniac, time addiction is assuredly anxiety-driven baggage.

Befriending time means nothing more than letting yourself become engrossed in what you're doing, focusing on this minute and not worrying about or contemplating future minutes. You're reading this book now, so why is your mind thinking of tomorrow's problems? Why do you need to know what time it is? See how long you can exist without wearing a watch; I let mine go in college and haven't used one since, and am as punctual as lunar phases.

Part of what's glorious about sleep is that while we're sleeping, time is decidedly unconstructed: it zigzags from present to past to future to past and even into bizarre states of nontime. Some call this schizophrenic, circular, or unorderly time, but isn't it enthralling?

As a North American, are you addicted to time? I learned my lesson on my first trip to Ireland in the mid-'80s, when cows still tottered down the middle of country roads. I was in Dublin, where the buses had published schedules, and I plotted out each line to determine how long it would take to get to my morning appointments.

All was well, until the bus driver jumped off the bus and started a long conversation with an old woman walking along the road, discussing, I think, her petunias. I looked on in shock as no one seemed to notice. Twenty minutes later he jumped back in and headed out, until after another several stops, he saw someone else he obviously knew and decided to have another extended chat, hopping back in his seat about 30 minutes later.

I finally asked the gentleman next to me, who was engrossed in his *Irish Times,* if this was standard procedure. He looked up and announced to an amused crowd, "Aye, yer girl here is an American. Always in a rush."

~ SIX SIMPLE WAYS TO BEFRIEND TIME ~

1. Stop wearing a watch.
2. Stop thinking about and checking every 5 minutes what time it is.
3. Eat your meals when you are hungry instead of at fixed times.
4. Go to bed when you are sleepy, and put time out of your mind.
5. Watch kids play and notice if they are obsessing about time.
6. Take one afternoon a month and do something you're passionate about: listen to jazz, go outside and draw, lie on the grass and look at clouds, go on a long hike, rent a stack of videos, garden. Resist thoughts about time. End only when you are done.

BEWARE OF YOUR
UNCONSCIOUS ATTITUDES

*In real life, I assure you,
there is no such thing as algebra.*
—FRAN LEBOWITZ

NOT FOR NOTHING IS INSOMNIA TERMED "THE loneliest club on Earth." It's lonely, yes, but insomniacs are also viewed as belonging to a type of insular club—a group of brave sufferers like chronic, low-level depressives and ultra-right-wing politicians. Bertrand Russell observed, "[People] who are unhappy, like [people] who sleep badly, are always proud of the fact."

It might sound strange to claim that something as draining as chronic insomnia or sleep disturbance could have any positive side benefits. However, take a good look at your thinking patterns, especially the unconscious attitudes you hold about your sleep problems—and how they interfere with, affect, and, yes, benefit, your daily life. These are called "secondary benefits" by sleep researchers.

Since these thoughts are subconscious, they won't readily pop to mind the first few times you call on them. However, once you get past the certainty that you have no unconscious attitudes or secondary gains from your troubled sleep life—how could you possibly?—do a little digging, and you'll be surprised at what you may find.

Here are just a few of the many possible secondary benefits:

I can't sleep so:

    I need a housekeeper.

    I can't get up early to exercise.

    I'm much more sensitive and less callous than others who sleep soundly in such a fallen world.

    I can't find a better job.

    My bad temper is understandable.

The way to uncover your unconscious thoughts is to pay attention to them and then write them down. In black and white, they inevitably look as destructive as they usually are. Use a journal to start a dialogue with the part of you that gets benefits out of your insomnia. Ask some tough questions and then listen to the answers. It's a similar process to dealing with stubborn weight issues: What are you getting out of being overweight? There are lots of answers to that question, as there are lots of answers to what you may get out of being chronically exhausted.

I remember a high school math teacher who let me have it when I blurted out why I was not understanding his questions: "I can't do calculus; I'm too fat!" Everyone thought that was funny and laughed—I was thin as rice paper at the time—but my teacher, rightfully, found no humor in it. He warned me to write that ridiculous sentence down on a piece of paper and carry it in my wallet until I graduated from college, which I did. From then on I always got A's in calculus and physics and all those fatless subjects.

We all have nutty thinking patterns, negatively reinforced bad habits, and self-defeating behaviors. It's part of being human. If you're serious about ridding yourself of sleep demons, these attitudes have to go. How unattractive to be seen as a bleeding-heart insomniac or wearing sleep problems on your sleeve as a badge of honor or excuse. Don't let your unconscious attitudes tether you to bad sleep; let them fly and get on with getting a good night's rest.

USE THAT JOURNAL

❧

*Be empty of worrying, think of who
created thought! Why do you stay in
prison when the door is so wide open.*

—RUMI

WHETHER YOU CONSIDER YOURSELF A WRITER
or not, journaling is an important tool in learning how to sleep. Most bad sleepers are notorious mind-swirlers, worrywarts, emotional resenters, hand
wringers, and plain over-reactors. Journaling—as opposed to
diary keeping—is a potent way to daily purge the tornado
of thoughts and feelings that overtake your mind.

A diarist from the time I could write, I've a garage wall of
notebooks jammed with childlike routine, youthful brag-
gadocio, and angst. Somewhere, though, I learned on my
own how calming writing about your true feelings is to the
central nervous system: my own way of dealing with lions
and tigers and bears. That lesson came with the shift from
diarist to journalist. This is an important distinction when
you start a journal in order to problem solve.

A dairy is a daily log of events and happenings. A journal
is a best book, a safe place to go and dump, explore, imagine,
invent, deposit, review, rework, whine, wallow, and generally
be every inch yourself. No masks. Who would the masks be
for? You write without judgment because no one ever sees

what you write or think. It's like a mirror, only you often don't know what you'll see until you finish writing.

And unless you have serious reason to believe your journal may end up with a grand jury, edit nothing, ever. If you don't feel a shudder at the thought of someone you know reading your journal, you're likely not using it to full potential.

There are lots of books specifically aimed at getting you started on your journal journey. If you're creative, daily journaling may be easier to begin than if you're a more pragmatic personality, but anyone can learn to use a journal to plumb a wild inner heart. Don't worry if you sound unhinged. That's the whole point: to find your hinge. Don't get nervous, because you don't have rules. That's what makes the journal process so testimonial; it's all truth, even if most of what you do as you write is tell lies. Certainly, that stage won't last long.

If you're intimidated by the thought of regular journaling, try this: For several weeks simply write for 15 to 20 minutes a day, morning or evening. Focus on keeping your pen moving at all times; this means no self-editing and resist the temptation to read what you've written when finished. Focus, instead, on how the process makes you feel once you're done. After a few weeks, your writing rhythm will gradually build on its own.

Journals are wonderful for all kinds of reasons besides learning to sleep better. But if you want to learn to sleep well, regular journaling is a powerful process. Often when I'm having trouble sleeping, I'll get up and write like a Fury—I've no idea about what until I read it the next morning.

Sometimes it even makes sense, and I often wake to find some quite beautiful and nervous poetry, none that I could write during waking hours. All I know is I feel as if a stone has been knocked off my shoulders when I finish—someone or something has heard my upset—and I'll think, "Well, it's OK, then," and soon fall asleep.

Just put anything you ever want to say, think, feel, or do in the book as often as you can—you'll get your unique rhythm and relationship going, and like any relationship, it will change and evolve over time. It's really about honesty, listening to yourself, and hearing yourself speak. And then relaxing. The only rule is: You need to do it consistently to earn results.

PRACTICE VISUALIZATION

*If you gaze for too long into the abyss,
the abyss also gazes into you.*

—FRIEDRICH NIETZCHE

JOHN LENNON'S SONG, "LUCY IN THE SKY WITH Diamonds," is über-visualization at its best: the freed mind meandering through a distorted and highly pleasurable mental photograph of your own making. Visualizations are dreams you consciously create in your own mind, and no matter that they may be filled with nonsensical images; this is your own private cinema, and you're director, writer, camerawoman, and star.

Learn how to visualize well, and you learn one ironclad technique to help yourself quickly relax and fall asleep.

The art of visualization goes by many names: "guided imagery," "mind photographs," "creative visualization." It simply means making, holding, and expanding a wonderfully distorted and vivid mental picture of whatever it is that gives you pleasure. Then focus on it slowly, deeply, and with great attention. What could be more fun and less difficult than that?

Imagination—that talent we all had an abundance of as children—is the key here, and if you're a natural right-brainer, you're in luck. There are no rules to this practice suffice that the images not be negative (no killing or blowing up your sleep disorder) but rather positive and bright. Pleasure, necessarily what brings you pleasure, is what you play with here.

To start, breathe deeply for several minutes and relax your muscles. Conjure up a handful of images that bring you pleasure, joy, a sense of safety, and feelings of deep relaxation. These will necessarily be personal to you. Pick one and hold it in your mind, using all five of your senses to explore the image in detail. What colors were there? What did it feel like on your skin? Remember smells, sounds, and tastes.

Live inside the image as best you can, for as long as you can, perhaps 10 to 15 minutes. If you like, you can tape-record your guided images and listen to them as you prepare to fall asleep.

A fun and easy trick to try as you get started: Visualize a word for a particular color—say, red—and then visualize it in silver. Or visualize words, such as *dark* in bright light, *rain* splattered in sunshine, *wood* filled with water. This helps you see how quickly your brain responds to image suggestions.

Practitioners say (and brain scans verify) that guided imagery works because, in terms of brain activity, picturing something and actually experiencing it are the same. The brain's visual cortex, which processes images, has a powerful connection with the autonomic nervous system, which controls involuntary bodily actions such as pulse, breathing, and stress response, and helps trigger the release of pleasuring hormones such as endorphins.

Visualization is used by many therapists for scores of self-improvement processes: goal setting, battling disease, grief work, relaxation, de-stressing, and weight-loss, among others. For sleep benefits, the best time to visualize is just before you drop off to sleep at night, during that yummy "twilight zone" between waking consciousness and sleep. Think of it as the mind-body's daily time of reverie and unbridled escape. In advanced stages, it's like playing with the id.

One thing researchers claim: Things that fall downward seem to be more sleep inducing than things that move upward. So fill your night dreams with banana-yellow Cadillacs circling down mountains, pink hankies falling from the sky, red-painted moons swinging lower and lower to Earth. Color, texture, and rhythm are all important elements.

For me, no matter what precedes it, I always end up at one of two well-remembered places: floating and sinking into the bright turquoise ocean around Anguilla, my favorite island, or sitting at the foot of the bed on the floor in Paris in late afternoon, eating a bowl of cereal and laughing out loud at *I Love Lucy*. But by then I'm usually unconscious.

~ VISUALIZATION ~

One of my favorite childhood books was C. S. Lewis's *The Chronicles of Narnia*. Aslan, the novel's huge brave lion, purred in my imagination until decades later when, as I struggled with sleep one night, he appeared in a lovely healing dream.

In it, two Aslans appeared: one towered over the scene as a massive warm ball of soft reddish fur, the other a block of white stone. I could climb neither until I suddenly saw myself, in aerial view, on the back of the furry Aslan, huddled in a fetal position in his comforting fur, sound asleep, safe and warm on his powerful back. I was deeply at rest.

I use this visualization when sleep eludes me because of emotional stress. Try it when you feel likewise: Imagine yourself atop the back of a strong, loving lion, curled up and secure, protected in his feathery, sweet fur. A safe place is always there for us to inhabit.

STOP INSOMNIA OBSESSIONS

MENTAL OBSESSION IS INSIDIOUS, AND WHEN it's related to insomnia, it's a Loch Ness monster. How many times during the day do you think a champion sleeper thinks about sleep? Probably none. A good sleeper? Maybe once or twice, with positive thoughts about how good it'll feel to sink into that goose down pillow.

How many times do you think an insomniac thinks about sleep during the day? You're probably in the ballpark if you guessed an astronomical number. For some reason, an insomniac's mind is tunneled on sleep—or the lack of—and chronic sleep conversations reign daily, either in endless internal monologue or with other unwitting listeners.

I was shocked once to hear my youngest brother suggest, "Listen, I know when you're not sleeping well because in response to 'How are you?' the first words out of your mouth are always the number of hours you slept. 'Well, I only slept 3 hours last night, from about 2 A.M. to 5 A.M. . . .'" I had no recall of any such rundowns. I was pushed into accepting my insomnia obsession, and into doing something about it quickly! Realize, first off, studies routinely conclude insomnia and lack of sleep for a night will neither kill you nor even negatively affect your performance the next day. The most it will affect is your mood and energy level, which may dip. You can live with this, certainly. Even if you didn't sleep at all for many days, your brain would make sure you got your deep-wave sleep when you did sleep (eleven sleepless night/days is the current world record). Part of your brain's survival function is to get more slower-wave sleep after a sleepless night, and it's something you don't have to be concerned with. Let it go.

Second, stop and listen to the thousands of automatic thoughts running through your mind daily. Tune in to the ones about sleep. If you follow the typical poor-sleeper profile, your sleep thoughts are chronically and boringly negative. Write them down for a week or two. When you feel ready for change, start psychically scratching out the negative thought and replacing it with a more intelligent, balanced, and less panicked thought. It's the same way you would try to change any bad habit.

Third, keep watch on your sleep-insomnia chatter throughout the day. It's become an oddly fashionable topic among women over age thirty, comparing stress and sleeplessness: "You wouldn't believe it, I was up with my daughter four times last night; I think I got about 2 hours of sleep." "I can beat that," you counter, barely registering the complaint, "I just got in from Chicago and had a layover in the airport. I haven't slept since Tuesday and I'm swamped!" Simmer down on your insomnia Olympics.

Maintaining tunnel vision about anything is a fruitless pastime, but when the obsession is about sleep troubles, stop wherever you are and think of something else, quick. It's the best thing you can do for your sleep.

WORK A WORRY BOOK

I'd rather sleep for three or four days
than do anything, so what happens?
I can't sleep at all. I worry about motor
tune-ups and the death of sparrows.
—CHARLES BUKOWSKI

A N INSOMNIAC'S BRAIN SCAN MIGHT SHOW something no scientist could verify and no pill could eliminate: there, clogged to one side, a clot of worries, clinging to whatever is currently on the worry channel, ruminating with racing redundancy. Does this sound familiar?

No matter the worries are intelligent and justified—aren't all worries?—this sapient little worry clot is going to make sure you have difficulty sleeping, no matter what. So how does a worrywart stop worrying?

Many sleep research specialists recommend writing in a worry book. Here, you take 15 minutes at the end of the day, perhaps an hour or 2 before sleep, and do absolutely nothing but good, focused, ejaculatory worrying.

It's simple enough. Buy a notebook or use index cards, anything that has enough room to write out a worry and a corresponding matching "action." To the left, write your current flagellation. On the opposite side, write down what your action is to eradicate this worry. Just be sure to always move from left to right—from worry directly to action—before you move on to another worry.

The salient question here: What is my plan of action for this worry? What can I do about this right now? What am I going to do about it tomorrow? This is hand wringing with a purpose, and it does work.

So if you're worried a freckle appears darker, or you look too fat in your jeans, you write in your worry book, "Will get more information about moles; query my sister about her new diet." It does not morph at 3 A.M. into, "Is that a lump? I must lose ten pounds by dawn." Another helpful idea is thematic worrying (much like tracking spent money). Where are the big fret-themes in your life? Work, family, health, money, children, friends, the future, persistent paranoias? If you have one pile that hogs all the cards or sheets, you know you're on to something.

Personally, I always tear up my worry notes immediately and throw them in the trash. I take great pleasure in the act of ripping them to shreds. However, many people like to have a keepsake notebook. It gives them a sense of structure, accomplishment, and power: These little melanomas won't metastacize when I sleep tonight, *danchachein*.

ACCEPT LARKS VERSUS OWLS

*Only dull people are brilliant at
breakfast.*
—OSCAR WILDE

DEAR BENJAMIN FRANKLIN, WITH HIS INFA-
mous dictum "Early to bed, early to rise makes a
man healthy, wealthy, and wise" branded the night
owl—the other half of the circadian lifestyle—as somehow
guilty of moral incertitude. However, if you want sanity in
your life, know who you are as a sleeper—a lark or an owl—
and simply accept your nocturnal biology and that of your
partner's. Leave the moral-indulgency clause alone. Larks
(those who spring from bed in the early A.M. with rabid en-
thusiasm) often do feel morally superior to owls (late-
nighters who burn energy into wee hours and are asleep
when the roosters crow). But research suggests genetics may
have a good deal to do with it.

Stanford University sleep expert Emmanuel Mignot the-
orizes that a mutation on chromosome 4—the clock gene—
plays a big role in your preference for morning or evening
life. Larks may seem gruesomely alert and perky in uncon-
scionable hours, and owls seem moody, a bit lazy, and rhythmically off balance, but neither is really true. Both larks and
owls show a normal circadian rhythm, but their cycles differ,
with owls' cycles peaking about 2 hours later than larks'.

This difference occurs in all physical cycles, including the daily rise and fall of body temperature and the increase and decrease in various hormones. It's simple biology.

It's best, of course, if partners are paired alike—two larks or two owls—because they innately understand each other's rhythms. But if you're not, the best course of action is to stop judging, being irritated by it, feeling or dispensing guilt—and, most important, trying to alter yourself. This last activity causes much useless stress.

Of course, if you're an owl and must wake early for work, you can accustom yourself to the circadian change. But if you still don't spring as peppy as other 5 A.M.'ers, even after years of trying, accept that *it's just fine*. (It's interesting, few larks ever feel the need to work themselves over into night owls.) Accept that your partner is just fine the way he is, too.

I know this one through experience. I am without a doubt a night owl; my mother, the ultimate lark. All during my school years I suffered in stunned silence as my mother would enter my room, fling open the drapes, and shout, "Good morning! Isn't it a beautiful day!" after having walked several miles, made breakfast, and had hours of productivity.

She'd regale me with stories from all the other larks she gabbed with on her walk. Asleep and unconscious, I'd hide until she shut the door. Why? Probably because I believed larkishness was better than owlishness, and who was I not to be taught this lesson? However, that all changed when I got to college and learned the art of late to bed, late to rise makes a wise woman whatever she wants.

HEAR YOUR SUBCONSCIOUS TALK

It is hard to fight an enemy
that has outposts in your head.
–SALLY KEMPTON

"THINK POSITIVE!" YOU MIGHT SHOUT TO yourself, which is just about the surest way to guarantee you won't. Myself, I need to already be in that sloganeering AA frame of mind to hear this kind of suggestion, where I now break from the past and embrace the phrases. "If you have lemons, make lemonade!" can be done.

Of all the tens of thousands of thoughts that race through your mind on a daily basis, how many could you remember correctly if some machine transcribed them? Probably only a handful. That leaves many thousands of thoughts—one of the most powerful forces that drive your mind, body, and health—without a director. Most people know what happens when wild horses are spooked and left without guidance: wholesale onslaught that can't be stopped.

If you want to take better control of your sleep, one of the surest ways is to start to control your thoughts and your thinking patterns. Hear what you (negatively) tell yourself about the world and your sleep. When you catch a negative thought (particularly about your sleep), quickly rephrase it into something more positive. Do this often enough and your mind learns how to make the changes automatically.

Taking control of thoughts, or more particularly the *kind of thoughts* that pervade your daily thinking, is a key element in learning not only how to sleep better but also how to function better as a human being—with much better health. Who doesn't want that?

Yet if you're like most people, you'll resist this think-positive self-improvement advice. There are seemingly good enough reasons: It's too difficult; Who wants to live with an occluded worldview?; I like the way I think, it makes me more sensitive; I was just born this way. You're probably well versed enough to know this is victim thinking: pessimistic thought patterns that are partly responsible for pressing you into your current sleep miasma.

Behavioral psychologists call changing your negative thoughts into more positive thoughts "cognitive behavioral restructuring," whereby you stay conscious of your thoughts and rearrange them into ones with more positive glow.

For example, you're driving and someone rear-ends you slightly. Do you breath fast, use creative finger puppetry, and immediately shout, "What an idiot!"? Or are you the optimist who first thinks, "I'm safe and the car is OK. No big deal." One of those thought scenarios is likely to sound strange and even slightly ridiculous to you, depending on your established thinking patterns.

Changing old negative thought tapes is a tough job. It can, in fact, be one of the hardest things you ever do. Here are some questions I ask myself when I first start seeing that slide down into the negative mind-bog:

Is this perception I have true?

Is it true to just me or to other people as well?

Am I trying to read minds, or should I ask what's going on?

What exactly am I angry (hurt, nervous, and so on) about?

Am I being oversensitive?

Will I care about all this in a month?

I often end up explaining the situation to myself as an adult would to a young child—amazingly, this lets you hear a more positive slant, as adults generally put positive spins on explanations to children.

And don't worry that you'll become the obnoxious person everyone knows who thinks so optimistically that everything they do is prone to wild exaggeration. Positive thinking isn't about self-delusion. It's about putting a gentler, sweeter spin on reality and letting go of some negative self-talk that nips at your brain like a bad verbal tic. With this one, your sleep will thank you in spades.

CREATE A SLEEP BIOGRAPHY

*Strange how things in the offing, once
their sensed, convert to things
foreknown.*

—SEAMUS HEANEY

REATING A SLEEP BIOGRAPHY, A RECORD OF
how you have slept—and those life circumstances
affecting your sleep patterns over the curve of your
life—is an important tool for overcoming chronic sleep disturbance. It's not something most people think about: How
well did I sleep in third grade? But if you walk slowly and
thoughtfully through your life, focusing on those events that
have led to the bad sleep habits you've formed, you'll find a
mass of information to explain what's lying underneath your
insomnia, much like cincture rings in a tree stump.

It's a fairly simple and even fun procedure. Take out a
piece of paper and create a long, straight, horizontal timeline. On the farthest left point, mark as far back as you can
remember (you can even take this too seriously and ask your
mother how well you slept as a baby: Was I a perfect sleeper
or a cranky all-night screamer?). Then moving toward the
right, plot how you remember your life chronologically by
age, school grade, job, city you lived in, marriage, children,
and other life stages.

Go back as far as you remember, and then ask yourself at various points:

> Did I sleep well or did I have sleep difficulties?
> When and why did the sleep problem appear?
> Was it ever resolved completely?
> Do I still carry some of that bad habit with me today?
> If yes, how so?

For instance, in second grade you started oversleeping badly and were often late for school. You had mononucleosis in college and started late-evening napping. A sibling's death, a parent's illness, a difficult move, a hospitalization, alcohol abuse in high school. Many people discover popping up all over their teenage and college years terrible sleep habits that were never quite eliminated.

Did you go through medical school or any educational program that noosed your sleep? Survived a traumatic life experience or assault? Have you slept well as a mother? (A dime for every woman who has told you she hasn't slept well since she had her first child.) Did marriage affect your sleeping habits? Perhaps when you shifted work to a home office, problems started to appear.

It's your timeline, so what shows up has meaning only for you. If you really did start lying awake at night stressing about life after you moved to Cincinnati at age twelve, and this nighttime worry habit never completely dissipated, this is significant information. Why? Because a part of that stressing child never got told, "It's OK. You can go to sleep now."

Take this information—now in a visual format—and circle all the bad habits in red. If you're like me, you'll see a kind of odd red slinky moving from left to right. Pay attention to what your bio says, and list out your bad sleep habits in order on a separate sheet of paper: erratic wake-up times, sleeping in on weekends, late-night eating, an alcohol or cappuccino nightcap . . . ?

You can either use this sleep biography to free yourself or pay a therapist to help you. Either way, pinpointing the development of bad sleep habits is important in starting to eradicate them. By naming them, seeing where and when they arrived in your life, and now moving on to get rid of them, you're on your way to better rest.

PERSEVERE,
AND YOU'LL GET THERE

If you start to take Vienna, take Vienna.

—NAPOLEON BONAPARTE

I T'S PROBABLY TRUE, YOU DIDN'T LEARN YOUR sleepless behavior overnight, and it's also a rather safe bet that you won't conquer it overnight, either. Eliminating sleep disturbances, especially if they're chronic, requires some exerted persistence—and intelligence—on your part. That means you'll need to be something of your own sleep specialist, psychotherapist, gumshoe, and best friend all at the same time.

You'll need diligence looking for clues and uncovering bad habits and discipline in setting goals to eradicate those bad habits, but also gentle understanding toward yourself. You'll need to give yourself a break in the routine when it all becomes too much, but also to persevere to your goal of deep, restorative sleep. Always keep that thought in the forefront of your mind: You can and will persevere to great sleep. Don't let anyone talk you out of it.

As much as you can, avoid listening to people who crow that once you learn your sleep restriction and deep breathing techniques, have your food and supplemental needs under control, eliminate internal poisons, correct all possible physiological causes, take care of snoring partners and yelling kids, and level out your hormones, all of a sudden you'll descend into Oz-ish poppy fields. Ultimately, that line of thinking only sets you up for failure. Surely, many women carry the insomnia ball for years, diligently moving closer and closer to their goal.

Remember, too, everyone has her own physiological structure, emotional makeup, unique life history, individual lifestyle, persistent problems and stressors. Imagining that millions of women can all use the same exact formulas to solve their sleep problems is like imagining death is going to pass you by, just because.

It's helpful to take a pragmatic approach to all the new information you have. Use your journal and lay out a specific, detailed plan, almost like a financial planner. You are then on a structured, forward-moving program, which always helps.

Record your progress and frustrations, and listen to your body. Always listen to your body. If what you're doing is causing problems, stop and reassess. There are many roads that lead to the top of the health-restoration mountain. Don't try to tackle everything all at once; go slowly and deliberately. Pick a few of the easier changes to start with, such as your sleep biography and bedroom air, and then move on to harder ones such as caffeine withdrawal and sleep and bed restriction.

As you see your progress, crossing possible problems and solutions off your list, you'll feel a sense of accomplishment and control—something important in the pursuit of good sleep. Don't stop until you find the sleep you want.

~ PAY OFF YOUR SLEEP DEBT ~

A gun can choose. A bullet has no choice.
—WILLIAM STAFFORD

If you think sleep is negotiable, secondary to your other daily duties and responsibilities, think again. If you need 8 hours of sleep a night but get up an hour early each day to walk the dog or do yoga, that equals a 7-hour sleep debt at the end of one week. That's 28 hours a month and 336 hours over a year. Over a decade or two, that simple 1-hour early morning act costs you many thousands of hours of sleep.

That's not to say one shouldn't have a dog or do early morning yoga. However, if your sleep is the first place you chop and slash to find extra time for your (sometimes necessary) activities, you're going to build up one nasty sleep debt.

Since everyone varies in how much sleep they need to function optimally, you need to know how much sleep you need, and then try to get it. How much sleep do you need? The rule of thumb is this: How many hours do you need to consistently wake up feeling refreshed without fatigue during the day? That's your sleep need.

If you need 9 hours of sleep to feel good, that means a far different schedule than if you need only 6½ or 7 hours per night. (And don't feel badly if you need more sleep than others; Albert Einstein left his global mark after reportedly slumbering up to 9 hours nightly.)

Sleep researchers claim even a minor sleep debt of 8 to 10 hours a week can affect your mood, motor abilities, hunger level, and energy. That's not a whole lot of wiggle room. Of course, the older you get, the harder it seems to withstand a big sleep debt.

Keep aware of how much sleep debt you run each week and try to get at least one good, long night to repay that debt. Studies show you can have a 30-hour or more sleep debt, and just one or two solid, uninterrupted nights of sleep can bring you back to nearly full payment on that debt.

It doesn't matter if lack of sleep is caused by work, family, leisure, charity, or any other wonderful thing. Piling up sleep debt—without paying the bank back—is a deleterious health hazard you want to avoid. Keep your sleep savings account full.

CHAPTER 5

FINE-TUNING THE BODY

EXERCISE

❧

Without discipline, there's no life at all.
—KATHERINE HEPBURN

I
T'S A WELL-KNOWN FACT: REGULAR EXERCISE IS essential to a healthy body and to a mind that's healthy enough to help get you to sleep. Do you exercise? Do you exercise regularly? Or do you sign up at the gym, buy the clothes, work out for two or three weeks, and then move on to other things? If you already maintain a consistent exercise program, great. If not, make the commitment to start one now—and just do it!

Pure and simple: Your body was meant to be used. Wonderful time-saving gadgets we have, but they're creating a population of muscle slackers that affect not only our health but our sleep, too. Since the rising and lowering of body temperature is a key factor in circadian rhythm—exercise raises body and brain temperature for several hours—exercise is a vital piece of the sleep puzzle.

Many insomniacs get themselves into a disconcerting cycle of sleeplessness, grinding low energy, lack of exercise, and thus even less sleep, especially stage 4 deep sleep. Anyone can talk themselves into paralysis about exercise: too tired, too busy. It's a universal procrastination. Only one person can change that cycle.

Exercise improves sleep for many reasons: It's a physical body and brain stressor, which is compensated for by deep-stage sleep. Exercise, of course, is at the same time a great body and mind de-stressor because it helps release built-up tensions and lactic acid in muscles; it vitalizes the nervous system, activates the endocrine glands, stimulates and strengthens internal organs like the heart and lungs, and—very important—improves mental functioning.

Walking is my personal preferred exercise—fast, slow, me-andering, any pace—at least 40 minutes twice a day, morning and early evening. If you have time for a quick 10- to 15-minute walk mid-afternoon, you'll see vast improvement in your late afternoon energy slump. Jogging, swimming, cycling, skipping rope, step classes, spinning, kickboxing, weight lifting, tennis, the Stairmaster, treadmill—our generation of sitters and ponderers has an endless supply of exercise vagaries. One must not forget to participate consistently.

Early evening is the recommended peak time for exercise aimed at improved sleep, about 3 to 4 (or even up to 6) hours before bedtime. Morning exercise, though excellent, won't directly affect your sleep, because your body temperature has already taken its fall. Refrain from exercise less than 3 hours before bed, as body temperature remains too elevated, making it more difficult to fall asleep.

Studies show the hormone epinephrine—a neurochemical linked with feelings of happiness and well-being—doubles in the body after 10 minutes of sustained exercise. Most people know exercise also stimulates the release of endorphins, the body's natural chemicals for alleviating pain. A healthful natural high.

The current temptation, though, is to put exercise on an obsessive treadmill of its own: we must exercise to help stave off fat, cholesterol, gravity, and incomprehensible mortality. However, try this: Think back to younger days when physical exercise was a seamless and alive part of your life.

We're not just talking about recess. Recall your young adult years: Did you get substantially more exercise than you do now? During high school and college, I thought nothing of a 2-hour prebreakfast tennis workout, an afternoon jog, a late-night cycle, all after navigating up and down miles of hills to class. Ballet classes, horseback riding, hikes, and swimming were on the weekends. Never once did I consider I was actually "exercising." I shudder to think what I'd feel like now, after even a couple of days of such expended energy.

Yet it's a good lesson to remember: I did what I did because I simply loved what I was doing. That's something to think about when you begin adding exercise back into your life.

STRENGTHEN
YOUR CIRCADIAN RHYTHMS

*Six hours of sleep for a man, seven for a
woman, eight for a fool.*
—Victorian Proverb

I F YOU THINK YOU SLEEP AND WAKE BECAUSE OF
things like alarm clocks, that's only partly true. Time cues
(called *Zeitgebers*), such as the sun, light, darkness, clocks,
and so on, strengthen and reenforce many of your naturally
occurring biological rhythms—specifically your circadian
rhythms—which run on an approximate 24-hour cycle.

Your circadian rhythm (from the Latin *circa,* "about," and
dies, "days") is cued most specifically to light—and your
sleep/wake cycle is set at about a two to one ratio, or 16
hours of activity with 8 hours of rest. You have nearly 100
biological and psychological circadian functions, such as
body temperature and hormone release, controlled mostly
by the hypothalamus, a deep and ancient part of the brain.
Thus, your circadian rhythm is an internal biological rhythm
guided by various external stimuli.

However, to complicate matters, this circadian rhythm, in
reality, runs on about a 25-hour cycle, so if all time cues are
removed—if you were placed in a darkened cave, for example, and let yourself sleep and eat when you felt like it—your
body would naturally shift an hour a day.

This is why it's so important to strengthen and maintain your circadian rhythm and sleep and wake cycle through use of a regular daily schedule—particularly with regard to light and dark—so your internal biological clock doesn't start floating, pulling you off course.

If sleep problems appear, reevaluate and strengthen the cues you send your circadian rhythm. At about the same time each day, make sure you get early morning sunlight, eat your meals, nap (if you take them), exercise, dim the lights, and retire for bed. Keep a tight string around your daily schedule, and your circadian rhythm will fall more easily back into place.

This circadian rhythm sleep/wake cycle is almost nonexistent in newborns, very strong in children, slower in teenagers and young adults, and by the thirties has regained a more natural rhythm, becoming faster in the elderly. This is why you probably had trouble going to bed and waking early in high school, college, and your early twenties and, if you're over sixty-five, probably fall asleep earlier and wake earlier than you'd like.

Where you are in the daily circadian cycle determines your energy level and alertness. People feel most sleepy in the early dawn hours, in the late afternoon, and close to bedtime. You'll also feel most alert in the morning and early afternoon and again in the early evening hours. This is a natural, biological rhythm, one that gets pulled off-kilter from varying sleep/wake patterns and loosened time cues.

Research shows it's also much harder to fall asleep at certain times of this daily rhythm. Termed the "forbidden zone," it's a period when it's extremely difficult, if not impossible, to fall asleep. This zone runs about 2 to 4 hours before your normal bedtime. Trying to sleep during these hours usually results in failure and frustration. Restructuring to a later bedtime is always best.

Light is your most critical circadian strengthener, though all your *Zeitgebers* are important. So the stronger your timed daily activities regarding light—an established wake-up time, that early morning walk, turning down bright lights in the late hours, a set bedtime—the better you'll sleep and feel.

SOOTHE YOURSELF WITH AROMATHERAPY

*Under the Moses of the incense you
have dozed off.*

—FREDERICO GARCIA LORCA

PERSONALLY, I THINK AROMATHERAPY AND women were made for each other. Ever notice the feminine need to smell nearly everything we come in contact with? What better way to bring balance, healing, relaxation, rejuvenation, and, yes, sounder sleep into your life than through beautiful, natural scent?

Aromatherapy is the blissful art of distilling essential oils from certain plants—there are about 300 that produce this type of oil—and using them to heal physical, mental, and emotional problems. The practice has been used medicinally since antiquity, was perfected in the tenth century, and given the name aromatherapy in 1928. Its power is both subtle and strong.

Indeed, the olfactory system is the only human sense that opens directly into the brain, into the limbic, or the more primitive, subconscious system. And since smell is the strongest of all your senses—10,000 times more sensitive than the others—it's not hard to understand the evocative power odor has on the human brain, sleep centers included.

Essential oils work not just through one but also through several of our physiological systems—olfactory, respiratory, and tactile—so the same essential oil has a wide variety of uses. You can use them in massage oils, inhalers, vaporizers, lamp burners, sprays, sachets, dropped into bath water, or dribbled lightly onto night pillows.

A large cast of essential oils can help maneuver you into sleep, so you have a broad pick if certain smells aren't to your liking. And remember, these smells need to be relaxing and satisfying to *you*. It doesn't matter what someone else says or what a book or aromatherapy sleep recipe indicates. If you can't stand lavender or clary sage (two good sleep helpers), don't try to make them work; simply try another oil or blend until you hit the right one for your brain and nose.

Sleep-enhancing essential oils include any of the following and work well alone or mixed into blends: basil, chamomile, clary sage, coriander, lavender, orange, mandarin, marjoram, melissa, neroli, pettigrain, rose, rosewood, tangerine, thyme, sandalwood, vetiver, and ylang-ylang. When in doubt, choose lavender, at least to start, as it's the perennial sleep favorite.

You can also use them as perfumes, dabbing them on your pulse points or between your breasts for more potency. As I've aged, I've noticed store-bought perfumes no longer sit well with my chemistry. They become too strong, too sweet, or too sour too soon. Yet one great thing about essential oils is that they remain stable; the scent doesn't change as you wear it, which means it won't give you a headache or keep you awake at night.

Since pure essential oils are aromatherapy's tools, try to use the highest quality oils available, particularly for something like insomnia. You'll need to store your oils in dark amber bottles in a cool, dry place, away from sunlight or heat; avoid leaving them in the bathroom. The oils are highly volatile and evaporate rapidly when exposed to air, so keep bottles tightly capped; never leave them uncapped for more than a few seconds. If properly cared for, most will remain fresh a year or longer.

A great trick you can use to check whether you have a bonafide, pure essential oil: Put a drop on a piece of paper. Pure essential oils evaporate, leaving no trace, whereas those in carrier oils leave an oily spot.

Anyone who walks past my room at night whiffs a beautiful blend of neroli and tangerine. My skin smells of neroli and marjoram, and on my pillow is a blend of Turkish rose, lavender, pettigrain, melissa, rose geranium, basil, and spikenard. And that's after I've taken a hot bath using this eternal aromatic blend: 3 drops lavender, 2 drops ylang-ylang, 2 drops grapefruit, 2 drops myrrh. It's not a replica of the fragrance described in the aromatherapy-drenched Canticle of Canticles—"He is a sachet of myrrh between my breasts"—but close enough for sleep, for now.

~ AROMATHERAPY ~

 Sleep pillows—or herbal sachets—have been given as gifts and placed under pillows since the colonial era. They've been used in Europe to induce sleep for centuries. Today, you can buy fanciful and expensive ones, but the handmade variety makes for a special treat. Also, they're easy to make if you want to save money. Here's a lovely potpourri recipe to try:

> 1 cup dried lavender
> 1 cup lemon balm (melissa)
> 1 cup dried orange or tangerine peel, ground
>   (or use essential oils)
> 1 cup rose petals
> 1 cup chamomile flowers

Combine all these herbs in a nonmetallic bowl and stir with a wooden spoon. Pour into a large empty sachet or small airy pillow case. Makes one 8-x-10-inch pillow. For a gift, decorate with fragranced ribbon or twine.

ENJOY A HOT BATH

When in doubt, take a bath.
—MAE WEST

REGARDING BATHS, I SUBSCRIBE TO MAE WEST'S thinking 110 percent. In my opinion, hot baths are God's gift to humankind. Here in the West it's, "I'll jump in the shower. Be out in a minute." Fundamentally unpreferable. Why would anyone want to rush the most pleasant part of the day?

Bathing is a reliquary of calm and rejuvenation, a succor echoing back to our amniotic state. It's also free; all you really need is water. And if you bring regularized—the key here is *regular*—hot baths into your evening, sleep will come more easily.

In other cultures—particularly in the slower-paced Mediterranean and Orient, with their Turkish *hamams* and Japanese *sentos* (public) and *furos* (private) baths—bathing is recognized as a ritual, something that promotes not only a sense of safeness when done solo but also a way to bind community and even generations together.

Many of the more choice female rituals, like belly dancing (an ancient female-fertility bath ritual) and wedding showers (where married females celebrated together in the communal bath, presenting the bride-to-be with gifts for her future baths) started right there in the tiled, steaming, sensual, relaxing, feminine hot bath.

Draw a warm (hotter than you normally like) bath, usually at least 100 degrees Fahrenheit, and soak no less than 25 to 30 minutes. You need to keep the bath continuously hot. This will cause a rise and fall in body temperature that makes it easier to fall asleep and stay asleep. Once your body temperature is raised, it falls once again as you lie down in a cool room. (Your body temperature drop post-bath occurs more quickly than it does after exercise.)

Be alert to the timing of your evening bath, taking it about 2 hours before bedtime. Some people like to steam and soak, cocoon in a Turkish towel, and then crawl into bed.

Though many people love to have scented candles flickering around when bathing, I always turn out all the lights and bathe in pitch dark. Wonderful. Try it this way at least once, and see if it suits you. Soaking in water, floating in the dark womb; we remember, even if we think we can't.

There are certainly numerous choices in bath oils, bath salts, scented soaps, loofas, pillows, bubble baths, and all kinds of bathing paraphernalia. Baths are now big business. Lavender, neroli, tangerine, patchouli, valerian root, lemon balm, rose, marjoram, and sandalwood oils are all excellent choices for a wind-down evening bath. Leave the stimulating ones, like peppermint, ginger, and eucalyptus, for a morning shower. Also, remember to pat yourself dry after your bath; don't vigorously rub, as this can be too stimulating.

Two good cost-busters: Instead of expensive pillows that routinely flatten out, roll a large towel behind your head, and rest your neck on it, which gives a good stretch. Also, you can buy inexpensive bags of plain sea salt at the grocery store and blend in a few favorite drops of essential oil. Baking soda and Epsom salts are two other bathing and soaking staples.

Here is a lovely before-bed bath mixture for relaxation and calm: Dilute into 2 teaspoons of sweet almond oil 9 drops of the following blend: 3 drops lavender; 2 drops ylang-ylang; 2 drops neroli; 2 drops tangerine. Add to bath water and swish well.

Experiment with what you like; a bath is very personal and not to be taken for granted. We have the freedom to partake in daily bathing, yet I know people who have not taken a proper bath in years. Bring hot bathing into your evening. You'll wonder how you ever lived without it.

NOTE: If you're pregnant, elderly, or have high blood pressure, hot baths are not advisable.

BREATHE

*Tension is who you think you should
be. Relaxation is who you are. Breathe.*

—JAPANESE SAYING

WHEN YOU BREATHE, YOU INTERACT WITH
the world at your most fundamental, intimate
level, literally foresting life to the planet. It's your
never-ending rhythmic connection to every living cell
through a perfect, balanced, interexchange of oxygen and
carbon dioxide. Perhaps, in part, it's the reason we're here: as
a kind of ecosystem photosynthetic gardener.

Breath control, at its core, is really about health—physical,
mental, emotional, and spiritual. If you have no connection
to your breathing—if it's simply on autopilot—it's likely
your breath is shallow, tight, restricted, and fast. Listen to
how you are breathing right now. Is this you? If you have
sleep disturbances, learning how to breathe slowly, deeply,
evenly, and unrestrainedly is a physiological practice that's
too important to ignore.

If you master no other relaxation technique to aid your
sleep, master the depth and regulations of your breath. Deep
breathing techniques are especially helpful in alleviating insomnia symptoms and promoting deep sleep if they're done
in bed, just before falling off to sleep.

Unlocking the bad-habit blocks that keep your breath fast and shallow helps calm down your central nervous system, pumps fresh red blood cells and oxygen to your body and brain, reinvigorates your internal organs, cools down your body, releases anger and frustration, and relaxes tense muscles. It's probably your one best all-around relaxation technique.

Watch little girls at play. Up until about puberty, young girls enjoy deep, wonderful "belly breaths." It's a fun, almost forgotten, female experience. You'll see their tummies moving in and out as they stand, perfectly unaware of what they'll unfortunately learn all too soon about the tight, chest-out posture, holding in one's stomach, small waists, and tummy-control pantyhose.

Relearning belly breaths is what you're after. There are two basic types of breathing: chest (costal), in which the rib cage lifts up and out and the air enters the upper rather than the lower part of the lungs; and abdominal (diaphragmatic) breathing, in which the diaphragm—a large, strong muscle—contracts to allow air to enter the lower lungs.

To discover if you're a chest or abdominal breather, when you lie down, simply look to see what is rising, your chest or your lower abdomen. Chances are, you're a chest-breather, but even if not, you can probably benefit from more concentrated, deep, lower abdominal breathing.

Take 10 to 15 minutes a day—preferably at bedtime or, better yet, in bed—and concentrate on breathing slowly and purposefully through your diaphragm. If you place your right hand on your chest and your left hand on your abdomen, you connect both your upper and lower body in a powerful way, as well as seeing when and how much your abdomen (and left hand) rises and falls.

Focus on your inhale, going as far and deep and slowly as you can, then exhale, slowly, evenly, deeply, until you imagine all the breath is pushed out of you. Keep the rhythm even, don't try to change it; let it move at its own pace. Just concentrate on becoming aware of your breath rhythm and its natural depth. Gradually, with practice and concentration, your breathing will move to its preferred, more relaxed state. Perhaps you can close your eyes and send some grateful thoughts to your lungs, those parachute-like organs that literally keep you alive.

To help you master good deep-breathing habits throughout the day, when tension and stress may conspire to shut them down, make notes to yourself and put them in your purse, on your computer, in your desk, on your bathroom mirror, on the refrigerator, above your bed, on your night stand. Only one word is needed: *breathe.*

DETOXIFY YOUR BODY

*That we are not much sicker and much
madder than we are is due exclusively
to that most blessed and blessing of all
natural graces—sleep.*

−ALDOUS HUXLEY

I F I COULD SUGGEST ONLY A HANDFUL OF THINGS
to help you get better sleep, one of them would be this:
Clean out your body, starting with your colon. This
might sound outrageous to the uninitiated, but cleaning
your bowel—the most important detoxifying organ in your
body—is critical for a clean body system, clean blood, and
getting fresh oxygen to the brain. A poisoned and toxic body
simply cannot sleep and rest properly.

I learned this the hard way. After decades of bad eating,
living in a polluted environment (in a city apartment next to
a garage), and many years of necessary daily medications, I
was so toxic that I literally woke up every hour. Almost
hopeless, I embarked on a journey that led to fasting; serious deep bentonite-and-clay colon cleanses; gall bladder,
kidney, and liver cleanses; and, most important, regular
colonic hydrotherapy.

After one year, I could sleep 6 hours straight without
waking, having changed nothing else in my sleep regimen. I

not only slept better, but I also felt reborn: I no longer felt like I was swimming underwater, with that mustard gas–like feeling that anyone whose body is toxically overloaded knows, and hates, well.

Colonic hydrotherapy is considered controversial by some. This, however, is what it entails: Colonic irrigation is the controlled passing of warm water through the colon via the rectum, using about 15 gallons of sterilized water. Pressure control and light abdominal massage help eliminate and cleanse the colon. The therapy helps remove built-up fecal matter and mucous, as well as tone and reshape often coiled and misshaped bowels. The process lasts about 45 minutes.

Think of your colon as a pipe. If old fecal matter is clogging the tube's sides, both elimination and absorption is impaired (the bowel is responsible for a portion of nutrient absorption). After much ill wear and tear, the tube can get misshapen, which only further hinders the elimination process.

Colonics are nothing new: ancient Indian yogins and the Egyptians regularly cleansed their bowels for better health. Europe still views the practice positively, as did the American medical establishment until the 1930s, when the era of instantaneous medicine and medication gradually took hold.

Your medical doctor may or may not agree with colonic hydrotherapy, and indeed, there are some medical conditions for which a colonic hydrotherapist should not administer a colonic. These include heart disease, ulcerative colitis, Crohn's disease, and advanced pregnancy, among others. So be sure to account honestly and accurately for your health condition if you seek to try a colonic. If you have any concerns, check with your doctor.

Health food stores and books are full of colon cleansing products, which give you a guide and a place to begin. For deeper cleansing, it's important to find a licensed colonic hydrotherapist and start a regular program. Know you'll find your way. The most important thing is that you commit yourself to the process—and follow through. Both your sleep, and your body, will thank you.

TRY HERBS

The most important fact about
Spaceship Earth: an instruction book
didn't come with it.
—R. BUCKMINSTER FULLER

THIS IS ONE INSTANCE WHERE IT'S GOOD TO feed your head. Nature provides all poor sleepers with natural, safe, and effective antidotes for disturbed slumber. Herbs and herb mixtures are decidedly effective in feeding your brain nutrients that help you relax and induce better sleep.

Before you take any herb or herbal mixture, learn all you can about those you think you want to try, make a list, and then contact your doctor—particularly if you take any medications. Contrary to popular belief, herbs are potent medicines that need intelligent structure and proper dosage. Certainly do not approach herbs with the attitude, "Oh well, I'll try anything once, and if it doesn't help, no harm done." Be cautious. Most herbal products are nonaddictive, but find out what's best for your situation, and dose accordingly.

Herbal remedies come in many forms, not just liquid or tablet. Each can be made into teas (steeping or soaking herbs in water for several minutes), infusions (longer steeping—10 to 20 minutes), decoctions (boiled rather than steeped herbs), tinctures (soaking an herb in alcohol, glycerin, or a mixture of water and alcohol, then straining), or extracts (filtering or distilling out some of the tincture's alcohol, making for more potency).

Tablets and capsules are made like conventional drugs: all liquid is removed from the extract, and the remaining powder is shaped into tablets or capsules. Injections of herbs enter the bloodstream as quickly as other injected drugs do and generally need the supervision of a qualified health practitioner. Oils, creams, and ointments are often used if the herb is not safely taken orally.

Here are some herbs used for centuries—and throughout the world—for sweeter, sounder sleep:

anise	berries	orange
bergamot	hops	passion flower
California poppy	kava kava	primrose
catnip	lavender	rosemary
chamomile	lemon balm	skullcap
fennel	marjoram	valerian root
gentian root	melissa	verbena
guta kola	mullein	vervain
hawthorne	oat	

Often you'll find proprietary blends of these herbs mixed with vitamins and minerals, particularly the B-vitamins. Personally, I've found strong success using herbs and herbal mixtures, such as valerian root and kava kava, as well as many prepackaged herbal sleep products found in health food stores.

With herbs, the idea is to know yourself, your own system, and your medical condition, and don't overdo. Consider these as nature's nighttime helpers. They're true medicines in many parts of the world. Why not use them?

GET A MASSAGE

*If an individual doesn't feel the
tensions, rigidities, or anxieties of his
body, he is denying the truth
of his body.*

—ALEXANDER LOWEN

CONTRARY TO POPULAR MYTH, MASSAGE IS A healing art—one of the oldest in the world—and not a kind of advanced sexual technique. In fact, regular massage is one of the best things with which you can bless your sleep, yourself, and your health.

Many people have come to lump massage with foo-foo pampering, which is far from what massage really is. Muscles tighten, knots build, and exercise can only affect and help you let go of so much. The warmth of live hands rhythmically loosening what's binding up your body is just pure, smart, preventative medicine.

What does massage ultimately do? Many things, but (second only to your breath) it helps you reconnect to your body and learn how to deeply relax, a crucial skill in your quest for good sleep. As we grow and age, we pick up and collect moments and memories of tension—a trauma here, a love lost there, an accident, a death of a loved one—and hold them in our bodies.

Although much of the mental and emotional tension such events created dissipates over time, the tension is stored in our muscles, causing us to stiffen and ache. Certainly, if you've been physically, sexually, and/or emotionally abused in any way, your body knows all about it and remembers every detail. Enter therapeutic massage.

All types of massage are available, a list that has grown primarily since the mid-1970s and Esalen. You can try Japanese shiatsu, Chinese acupuncture, acupressure, polarity therapy, craniosacral therapy, deep muscle massage, Rolfing, Reichian therapy, sports massage, Swedish massage, La Stone therapy, the Hawaiian Lomilomi, as well as energy-balancing treatments such as Reiki, aura balancing, chakra clearing, and Healing Touch. The list seems endless. And the search is fun, too.

Key is your choice of masseuse. You're letting this person not only into your personal space but also all over your body; and when feelings erupt, as they often do if you partake of routine bodywork, you need to feel very comfortable with your masseuse. Word of mouth is the best reference, and like psychotherapy, there's a lot of trial and error in the beginning. What's good for one person may not work at all for another.

Here are two pointers: First, try to find a massage therapist who's skilled in many different approaches, who can blend and adjust a massage to your needs and body. Someone who only does deep muscle massage is limited, and there are simply too many good, multiapproach masseuses available.

Second, try the delicious Hawaiian Lomilomi if you can find it. There's no real way to describe this massage, where

the masseuse never actually uses hands but only arms and el-
bows. Call different massage schools and ask for referrals in
your area. Without question, this is one massage you won't
quickly forget.

~ MASSAGE ~

Here's a fun, hale-ful reflexology trick used at spas. Gather
a dozen or so Chinese river rocks (you can buy these small
black stones in many home and garden stores). During
an afternoon relaxation break, preheat ten stones in a hot
towel and wrap one or two in a cold towel. Place eight
warm stones between your toes; lie down and put two
warm stones under you at the lower part of your back and
one or two cooled stones on your forehead, between your
eyebrows. Cover your eyes and forehead with a cool towel
or an aromatherapy eye mask. Breathe deeply and evenly
for 15 minutes. Your muscles will relax as your mind
unwinds.

EXPERIMENT WITH BACH FLOWERS

❧

Over a sky of daisies I walk.
—FREDERICO GARCIA LORCA

FOR NEARLY A CENTURY, MILLIONS OF PEOPLE
worldwide have used Bach Flower Essences to
treat illness. It's a safe, nonaddictive, no-side-effect
method—one that has the true claim of being "all natural."
Bach Flower Essences are plant essences used as tinctures to
correct disharmony between the soul and mind—fears, anxieties, obsessions, worries—that British physician and home-
opath Dr. Edward Bach believed are the root cause of illness,
including insomnia.

There are thirty-eight Bach Flower Essences (plus one
composite essence, Rescue Remedy®), and ingestion of the
essence transforms the negative mental attitudes associated
with disease into positive ones. This, in turn, allows the
body's own immune system to fight illness and stress in peak
condition.

Take a few drops of the selected Bach Flower Essences
(which come in liquid form and are available at most health
food stores) under the tongue, or put them into water or
fruit juice and sip as a beverage throughout the day. It's quite
simple. You can repeat treatment over a course of several
weeks, during which time a feeling of emotional well-being
should gradually increase as your sleep improves.

Here's the tough part about the essences. Each essence targets a particular personality disharmony. There is no one essence for "insomnia" or "not enough sleep," but various different essences are targeted to personality flaws underlying the sleep disorder.

So for one person, "holly" may be required (this tincture is for someone filled with jealousy, hate, mistrust, and anger toward other people). For another, "agrimony" (for someone who hides worries behind a cheerful, smiling face and dodges conflict) would be appropriate. Each essence comes with a list of questions to determine which tincture seems most descriptive of your personality.

When you first read the descriptions, it may seem they all apply to you. However, upon closer inspection you'll notice certain ones stick out and irritate you more than others. Take special note of these. The essence descriptions of personalities are unflattering and thus require rigorous honesty to work. It's suggested that you have a close friend help choose the flowers that best match your personality, but that she do so secretly, by buying and pouring them directly into your mixture. You might take this advice.

Skilled practitioners help diagnose quickly and correctly, but since the system is inexpensive ($10 per essence), and no harm occurs if you take an essence that's not your correct match, you might want to try a few yourself first. Only be honest.

DO A SLOW DANCE

❧

*Nothing is more revealing than
movement.*

—MARTHA GRAHAM

ANCERS KNOW HOW RHYTHMIC BODY
movements positively affect mental and emotional
health. Just the slow, breath-full pull of muscles,
the practiced movements to music and time, help dancers
inoculate against stress and negative outside influences. It's
called grounding, and dancing is, like Irish poet Seamus
Heaney says, "like rowing the steady earth."

Slow dance is a Westernized version of the famed Chinese *tai chi ch'uan* exercises. (*Tai chi* is another excellent
movement exercise used to help reduce stress and learn
proper breathing, with great sleep benefits.) Slow dance is
simply a free-form modern dance routine, done in about
the same rhythm as a Gregorian chant—in other words, as
slowly and fluidly as possible.

The result is a combination of gentle, flowing movement
with stretching and deep breathing.

Slow dance is almost the exact opposite of the popular
"ecstatic" dance, where people gyrate from inner cues to
varying changes in loud global beats. Here, one rhythm is
used, and it is slow and soft.

Don't worry if you think of yourself as three-footed. No
one is going to see you, and no one is going to judge you.

This is just movement that flows out of your inner rhythm, set to music, to help you settle down and hear your own heart beat.

Like belly dance, another decidedly feminine dance, slow dance is best done barefoot. Outside—day or night—is preferable. Wear loose clothing or yoga workout gear, and make sure your headphones stay put without use of your hands, which need to be completely free. That's all you need. You can, of course, dance without music, just using your own internal rhythms.

Concentrate on the area in the lower abdomen about 2 inches below the navel. This is the hara—a term taken from Hatha yoga—and focusing there instead of constantly inside your head helps kindle physical confidence.

Then, just move. No more rules than that. Bend, reach, tremble, stir, vibrate; just move as if no one is watching, because no one is. This is not the same as going on a retreat and becoming a jaguar in a movement class—though if that's what your body feels like doing, why not? I usually slow dance outside at night, under the moon and stars, listening to classical and chant rhythms.

It takes about 20 minutes to thoroughly wind down, and if you keep breathing, you'll feel like you've awakened from a deep massage, deep prayer, and a symphony all at once. If you don't block anything and let whatever dwells in your subconscious rise up, you'll sometimes get profound emotion out of the dance as well.

This, I think, is a lovely and simple addition to any woman's relaxation and wind-down routine. And a good way to practice loving your own beautiful body.

KEEP A SLEEP LOG

❧

Details are the annoyance of life, but
also the way things become beautiful.
—ANONYMOUS

DON'T WORRY, THIS IS NOT THE SAME AS writing down every morsel put in your mouth or every penny spent during the last month. (Congratulations to anyone who has ever finished those exercises.) A sleep log is similar, though, and relies on the same principle: your sensory and memory perceptions are often highly poor indicators of what reality really is. Some people are so stubborn, they'll believe they didn't sleep a wink when, in fact, they slept for hours.

When you take a few minutes to jot down the particulars of your sleep patterns and mental thoughts, interesting and sometimes electrifying insights appear, seemingly spontaneously. Few of us are aware of our quirky thoughts or behaviors until we see them written down in black and white.

Use a notebook, or loose sheets of paper, anything large enough to keep bi-daily tabulations. It's basically two lists: What I Did During the Day (do this one at the end of the day, before you go to bed) and What Occurred Last Night (do this right when you wake up in the morning). You can do them quickly, probably in 1 or 2 minutes. Keep them together, and at the end of several weeks, see if any topical patterns emerge.

Some sample night questions to review the day:

Did I take a nap?

When did I exercise?

Did I feel fatigued or sleepy during the day, and if so, when?

What did I eat or drink, and if so, when?

Did I worry about sleep during the day?

What were the days' stressors, and when did they occur?

For morning interrogation about the previous night:

Did I take sleep medication?

What time were lights out?

When did I actually fall asleep?

Did I wake up during the night, and how many times, and for how long?

What were my sleep-related thoughts during the night?

Did I wake up with an alarm?

What time did I wake up?

What time did I get out of bed?

Look for, as well, things like green tea at 9 P.M., an argument with your spouse just before bedtime, the fact you skipped exercise five days during the week, the little bowl of ice cream just before lights out. Do these things affect sleep? For lousy sleepers, you bet.

Keep a log like this for two to three weeks, which is long enough to start seeing patterns appear. Use it as if you were your own sleep specialist tracking down those bad habits that cause fitful nights, and start eliminating them. This type of informational record is also extremely helpful when you visit a physician or other health-care professional for aid with sleep problems.

USE PHOTOTHERAPY

Who plans suicide sitting in the sun?
—ELIZABETH SMART

HOW MANY HOURS A DAY DO YOU GET SUN-light—nature's best sleep *Zeitgeber* (time cue)? If you're like the average North American, that number is a dismal 1 hour per day. Unless you work outside, you probably fill your sunlight quota with a sunglass-shaded trip to the car and to work and back. Maybe you toss in an early morning walk, though with today's concern about the sun's damaging UV rays, those are probably hatted and sunglassed, too.

Sleep-and-mood specialists are asking, Where has all the sunlight gone? Theories suggest that the extreme lack of natural daily sunlight exposure is affecting the general population with increasing mood and sleep disorders, indeed creating a kind of Prozac nation. By simply getting more sunlight during the day, you positively affect and protect your sleep system.

Before Thomas Edison invented the artificial light bulb, sunlight and true darkness (not street-lighted darkness) were the time cues for your body's natural sleep rhythm. Sunlight meant the rise of body temperature and a decrease in melatonin to promote wakefulness, and darkness meant the fall of body temperature and an increase of melatonin to promote sleep. Relatively simple.

Enter artificial light, and people now stay up way past sunset—often 5 to 7 hours. (The light bulb has also made the 24-hour workday possible.) This shifting of ancient circadian rhythm has effects on your hormones, including cortisol, your stress hormone, which affects your ability to rest and sleep properly.

And if you work indoors in a fluorescent-lit building, ouch. You're getting about 500 luxes of light (a lux is equivalent to the light from one candle), compared to 10,000 luxes of sunlight at sunrise and 100,000 at noon on a bright summer day. The inference here is that to your brain, you are spending the entire day in darkness.

Light therapy, or phototherapy, uses natural or artificial light to treat depression and sleep disorders. (If you have bipolar illness, you should not use artificial light therapy. Check with your physician.) Natural, full-spectrum sunlight is the best form of light to use, but sometimes during the low-light winter months, when seasonal affective disorder (SAD) can appear, simulated sunlight from light boxes is the treatment of choice.

A light box normally has a 10,000 lux capacity, and if you suffer from SAD, practitioners usually recommend sitting from 15 to 40 minutes in front of the light box at set early morning and late afternoon hours. This "tricks" your brain into thinking it's really summer, with longer daylight hours.

Some other simple things you can do if you want to prolong light hours during the day: Open your drapes right when you wake up, and keep them open until dark; take an early morning and late afternoon walk, and don't wear sunglasses early in the morning and at sunset.

It's a simple and pleasurable thing to do, and not just for better sleep. Get out in the sunlight, and let your eyes drink it in.

~ COLOR THERAPY ~

To some, human beings are, in fact, "beings of light"—each one built of energy of various wavelengths akin to the vibrations of each color. Sound a bit New Age-y? You don't have to understand nor even subscribe to this theory to know that light and color are healers for all kinds of physical and emotional mind-body troubles, including sleep.

According to energy medicine experts, each organ and gland corresponds harmonically with a certain wavelength of light. Ailments correspond with a deficiency of a color, and "light bathing" is adding the correct color, typically through the addition of light. It's called "heliotherapy"—and it seems to work for many people. The best color of light is full-spectrum sunlight, experienced while wearing as few clothes as possible. Remember the great feeling you had after a long day at the beach and how well you slept at night? The sun is a universal healing color.

Good colors to consider for sleeplessness: pink, green, indigo, turquoise, blue, violet, and/or purple. A simple method is to buy a light bulb of the target color and sit near it, with as much skin exposed as possible. Also, buy cellophane in the color and place it on a skin-diver's mask, or wear colored sunglasses, inside or out. Even several minutes a day can have a good effect. However, the sun is available to everyone, and it's free and simple. Soak it up. Just remember your sunscreen.

TAKE A CONSTITUTIONAL

❧

The woods are lovely, dark and deep.
But I have promises to keep.
And miles to go before I sleep.
And miles to go before I sleep.
—WALT WHITMAN

WHEREAS IT'S NOT A GOOD IDEA TO WALK FAST or exercise heavily late in the evening, a short, relaxing "constitutional" is really a wonderful way to slow down, unwind your mind and body, breathe deeply, be enveloped by nature, and listen to nighttime sounds. It used to be called an evening stroll, I think, something akin to sitting out on front porches with the neighbors at dusk. I promise you, this one is addictive.

Isn't it surprising how intense people are about their morning runs, walks, and exercise? And that's fabulous. But just because calories aren't burned at a furnace pace doesn't mean slow walking isn't productive walking.

You can choose to go it alone or with a partner—either way, it's a time set aside to look at your surroundings, maybe say a prayer, let your mind wander, and be silent while you move your body at a slower, easier, more relaxed pace. There's something about the dark night and crisp air, about stars and ingratiating crickets that intimates: There's nothing here to get tied up in knots about; just breathe, move, and gaze.

It's great if you get into a timed routine for your constitutional, making it part of your bedtime routine. Of course, where you live—and the weather—are factors in how many months of the year this is reasonable. Luckily I live in clement weather, but I do know friends who take their constitutionals seriously enough to plow out in the rain or snow.

Think of water, the substance that makes up about three-quarters of our body. When confronted by a flat surface, it meanders by nature, invariably taking the roundabout approach. You can do the same on your nightly constitutionals, either walking the same path nightly or indulging in some wanderlust; just make sure to keep it slow.

How often is up to you. Once or twice a week is good, but every day, at the same time, if possible, is perfect. If it's safe enough in your area to walk at night alone, great; if not, don't despair. Do it as late as you feel safe. Sunset is a fruitful time to walk without worry about pulse rates.

Nighttime, after all, is when nature is slowing down, turning inside itself for rest and a different kind of rhythm. Get into the habit of tuning in to this slowed twist of time, and you'll notice the same plants that looked bright and vibrant just 12 hours earlier really do look more subtle and subdued. Ever wonder why monks and nuns often walk peacefully before retiring? Here's your answer.

STRETCH AND BREATHE WITH YOGA

❦

*Blessed are the flexible for they shall
not bend out of shape.*

—ANONYMOUS

GOOD, LIMBER, PLIED LIMBS AND BODIES ARE in a much more relaxed state than tense, tight, and rigid muscles, would you agree? Why then do so many people not take the time to limber up and stretch their muscles and diaphragm before bed?

It only takes about 10 or 15 minutes to do a good stretch-and-breathe routine. Ballet or runner-type stretches are fine, or you can use the more ancient stretching and balancing yogic poses. Either way, the benefits far exceed just a better night's rest.

Myself, I use yoga postures both in the morning and before bed. Believe me, there's nothing like a few of those pure, undiluted yogic breaths—which come every blue moon—to keep you committed. Certainly, yoga is an antidote to daily, chronic stress, and those who speak of it with religious fervor are disciplined devotees who don't dabble. But for sleep purposes, one needn't be a yogin. Indeed, the wonderful thing about yoga is that you can choose your level and interest, yet still reap benefits.

Yoga is the Sanskrit word meaning "union" or, more literally, "yoke." There are many branches of yoga; the most commonly practiced Western branch, Hatha yoga—the yoga of force—is the practice of physical postures (called *asanas*) and breathing techniques (called *pranayama*.) It emphasizes physical strengthening and purification and works to restore and heal the body, helping it function at optimal level. There are many good classes to help you get started and to ensure that the poses and the breathing are done properly.

To use Hatha yoga postures to help ready you for sleep, wear loose clothing, remain barefoot, and find a quiet, warm place. Come into each position slowly, hold it for a few breaths, and come out of it slowly. Never force your body to move into or hold a position that hurts. Rest in between postures, registering the effects on your system. Breathe slowly and evenly, and always focus on your breath. Continuous concentration on your breathing throughout each posture is the key to yoga.

These are the eight poses I use daily (I only do the Corpse pose at night) and are particularly good to help women limber-up and relax: Child's pose, Up Dog, Down Dog, Ragdoll, Butterfly, Seated Forward Bend, Inverted Waterfall, Corpse pose.

CHILD'S POSE – Sit on your heels and lean forward so that your chest rests on your thighs and your forehead touches the floor. Relax your arms at your sides, palms facing ceiling. Take at least six full breaths, feeling your back swell and contract as you inhale and exhale.

UP DOG – Lie facedown on the floor, hands on the floor at your waist, fingers pointing forward. Legs should be parallel and a few inches apart, with the soles of your feet facing the ceiling. Slowly straighten your arms to lift your torso and hips off the floor. Looking straight ahead, lift your chest and let your shoulders roll back. Hold this position for at least six breaths.

DOWN DOG – Get on your hands and knees and curl

your toes into the floor. Lift your hips toward the ceiling and straighten out your toes so that you're balancing on flat feet and palms; your fingers should be pointed forward. Keeping your legs straight, arch your back gently and press back through your arms, letting your head relax toward the floor. Hold for a minimum of six breaths.

RAGDOLL – Stand with your feet six inches apart, feet pointing forward and parallel. With knees relaxed, bend forward at the hips, torso toward the thighs. Bend your arms, holding the left bicep with the right hand; rest the left hand on the outside of the right elbow. Press your hips toward the ceiling to feel a stretch in the back of the legs. Hold for six breaths, then slowly roll up to standing, chin to chest.

BUTTERFLY – Lie on your back with your legs lifted and your hips against a wall. Bring the soles of your feet together, and with your hands against your knees, press your legs open as far as you can comfortably. Hold for six breaths.

SEATED FORWARD BEND – Sit with your legs stretched forward, feet touching and toes pointed toward the ceiling. Bend forward and gently touch your toes with your fingers. If you can't touch your feet, reach forward toward your toes as far as you can. Hold for six breaths.

INVERTED WATERFALL – Lie on your back with your legs lifted and your hips against the wall. Lift both legs to a full straight-up position. Pull toes forward, perpendicular to the wall. Hold for six breaths.

CORPSE POSE – Lie flat on your back, with arms extended to both sides, palms facing slightly up, feet loosely falling to the sides. Relax all muscles, close your eyes, and breathe deeply for 10 to 15 minutes.

Hatha yoga makes us sensitive to our bodies—where we are weak or strong, and also where we are flexible and inflexible. (You can also translate this into your daily life; they often parallel.) The postures also help cleanse the blood, lightly massage and stimulate the internal organs, affect glandular activity, increase metabolism, and improve digestion. And because yoga is so calming to the central nervous system, you're much more relaxed and at ease in your own body. A good thing, for both you and your slumber.

~ SEX ~

Drop lower and lower into the deep river of
sex and I'll kiss you more.
—JOAN LOGGHE

Sleep experts seem to agree: Sex used as a soporific is a wild card. True, a good sexual experience just before sleep can promote a sense of relaxation and a luscious warm glow. A less-than-good or a bad sexual experience, on the other hand, promotes just the opposite. Add to this mix the exhaustion of parenting, work, life in general, your monthly cycle and/or hormonal changes, and using sex as a sleep aid is no sure thing.

It's not news that women and men can approach love and sex differently, sometimes seemingly from different parts of the playing field. And although you may need more stimulation than a man to climax—including prolonged foreplay, caressing, and kissing—once aroused, you're capable of sustained orgasm, while he must wait for a sexual recharge.

As a woman, this leaves you vulnerable regarding sex and sleep. If the encounter is rushed, and your heart, let alone your pelvis, hasn't opened up enough to truly be released, frustration reigns as you look at your probably sleeping partner, you wide awake, your body still aroused and ready for more talk and/or sex.

This isn't always the case, of course, and making love has been used for centuries as a way to get to sleep. But it might help to know that a sleeplike brain-wave pattern immediately postorgasm is a documented phenomenon throughout the male animal kingdom. It might lessen your frustration and resentment toward your partner—two unhappy feelings if you wish for peaceful sleep—if you see it as a physiological inevitability.

Sex and sleep cycles throughout the night are also linked. During each period of REM sleep, both you and your partner's erectile tissues (penis and clitoris) are stimulated: it's during REM sleep that both men and women have nocturnal erections and orgasms. You have about four such sexual stages during the night. That's why in other cultures, particularly the East, sex is routinely engaged in not at night, before all these REM stages have occurred, but in the morning, when you are fresh from your REM-stimulated sleep. You can, if you time yourself right, awaken during the final REM stage, which usually occurs right before wakening; some sex counselors claim this improves and heightens sexual intensity.

If you don't have a regular sexual partner, masturbation produces the same climatic release, physiologically speaking, which is simply good for your body and health. My hope is that knowledge has helped you overcome guilt regarding self-love, but if not, consider that guilt is not a sleep-conducive feeling, either. So regarding sex and better sleep, it's really your personal call.

KNOW YOUR SLEEP POSITIONS

*When I am alone, I can sleep crossway
in a bed without an argument.*

—ZSA ZSA GABOR

DO YOU KNOW WHAT POSITION YOU REGULARLY take up in bed when you drop off to sleep? According to sleep researcher, Dr. Samuel Dunkell, the position you choose in bed each night echoes the way you deal with your daytime waking hours. Invariably, you often sleep as you live. These chronic sleep positions can affect your sleep, positively and negatively.

A highly private matter, choice of sleep position, the theory goes, gives insight into not only sleep patterns, sleep history, and sleep difficulties but also personality traits and those of your sleep partner's. And if applicable, it can even delve into hidden subconscious secrets buried in your relationship.

Tonight, when you climb into bed, pay attention and observe what position you spontaneously assume to make yourself feel most comfortable at just the moment when you decide to fall asleep. This is termed your "preferred sleep position." What is your preferred sleep position, and has it changed over the years? Has it had an effect on your sleep efficiency, or is it causing discomfort or pain? If your preferred position affects your sleep negatively, teach yourself to sleep in another, more sleep-promoting position.

There are four basic individual sleep positions:

1. In the *prone* position, the sleeper lies face down on the stomach with arms extended and bent, usually framed above the head. People—and I am in this group—who regularly sleep in the prone position tend to have strong compulsive tendencies in their personalities.

2. The *royal* position is the geometric opposite of the prone position. The royal sleeper lies supine, fully on the back, with arms slightly akimbo at the sides. It's an open, vulnerable and expansive position, and these individuals are said to display self-confidence and self-involvement.

3. The most common position, the *semi-fetal,* has sleepers lying on their sides with knees slightly bent, one arm outstretched above the head, the other resting comfortably on the opposing upper arm to cradle the head. Conciliatory, compromising, nonthreatening, nonshakers. This is claimed by sleep experts to be the optimal sleep posture position.

4. The *full-fetal* is the characteristic womb position. Sleepers lie curled on their sides, with knees pulled all the way up, heads bent forward. Usually a pillow or blanket mass is centered at the stomach. These sleepers are highly emotional, sensitive, artistic, and have intense one-on-one relationships. Oddly, it's found that women who sleep in this position normally have heightened capacity for multiple orgasms.

Couples' sleep positions are equally telling, with the lovely *spoon* position most common for partners in the first three to five years together. Here, both partners lie on the same side facing the same direction, one behind the other, a set of spoons curved in the night.

The *bridge* position has the domineering partner placing a leg over the body of the sleeping partner, using the royal position. The *freeze maneuver,* each with their back to the other, pulled over to separate sides of the bed, shows anger and distance. The *umbilicus* position is a sort of separated spoon with one partner reaching over to lay hands on the other for security. There are the *shingle, reverse shingle,* the *hug,* the *switch,* and lists of others. You alone get to choose which one sends you into the deepest state of sleep each night.

RESTRICT YOUR SLEEP

❧

*Sleeping is no mean art: for its sake one
must stay awake all day.*
—FRIEDRICH NIETZCHE

As A SLEEP-STRUGGLER, IT'S LESS AGGRAVATING imagining that all of the extra time you spend in bed gives your body good rest. The Germans call it *Schlimmbesselrung:* an intended improvement that only makes matters worse. Sleep therapists loudly claim this extended bedtime routine is pure false hope.

In fact, spending more time in bed than your body needs for sound sleep dilutes the sleep process: it makes it harder for you to fall asleep, increases the number and length of nighttime awakenings, and makes your sleep much more shallow, with much more stage 1 sleep and little delta or slow-wave sleep.

Why? It's like pouring a gallon of water over a larger surface; it spreads out thinner and more shallow the more room it has. The same is true for sleep and time; extend your hours in bed, and the shallower sleep is less restorative. You'll wake up more tired and fatigued than before. The vicious cycle begins. You're sleeping and feeling worse, so you kick up your time in bed, going to bed earlier or waking up later (particularly on weekends), and start taking naps. You can see where this is headed.

Sleep restriction is the therapy used to restore the proper sleep-time equation, or what's called sleep efficiency. What you are doing is compressing and confining your time in bed to the hours you actually spend asleep. Everyone can do the mathematics here: simply count the number of hours you are actually *asleep in bed* during a 24-hour period. If it's 6 hours and your goal is to sleep a full 8 hours, pick a wake-up time, say 7 A.M., and count 6 hours backward. Voilà, you've identified your new sleep-restricted bedtime (1 A.M.), wake-up time (7 A.M.), and eventual goal time (11 P.M.).

Here, this means you'll not turn out the lights until 1 A.M. When you've slept straight through the night from 1 A.M. to 7 A.M., move your bedtime up 15 to 30 minutes (12:45 A.M. or 12:30 A.M.) each night until you sleep straight through. Continue moving bedtime up the same number of minutes until you reach your full 8 hours of sleep.

Accept that your body will rebel, you'll feel inordinately tired at night waiting around till all hours to go to bed, nothing much is fun, and isn't this ridiculous? Or if you plan it the other way around (earlier bedtime) and get up at 4 A.M., what in heaven's name is of value at 4 in the morning?

However, once you set a bedtime and wake time, stick to it as if your income depended upon it. It's one of the best sleep habits you can acquire, and you'll feel triumphant when you finally sleep well, sleep straight through the night, and wake up rejuvenated.

CHAPTER 6

SOOTHING
THE SOUL

REDUCE ANGER AND RESENTMENT

*I'll go to sleep if I can; if I cannot, I'll
rail against all the first-born of Egypt.*
—SHAKESPEARE, *AS YOU LIKE IT*

NGER IS THAT PLACE DEEP INSIDE YOU, FED since childhood, that searches out and spotlights all that hurts and makes you feel unsafe. A psychologically necessary emotion, anger—and its overdosing corollaries, resentment, hostility, rage, if left to run wild—is nonetheless one of the most damaging emotions you can experience. Without question, anger and its friends are all sleep-eroding poisons.

It's helpful to know what anger is and is not, what it can and cannot do, for and against you. In its rightful place, anger lets you know when you're being hurt, demeaned, treated unfairly, threatened, blocked from an important goal, or the recipient of someone else's anger and ill intent. You might also experience righteous anger toward injustice and global wrongdoing that mobilizes you for positive change.

At its most fundamental and often subconscious level, you get angry over something you perceive as a loss. You rant in your subconscious, a holdover from hyperdependent infancy and childhood: Someone should have been there to see me, hear me, protect me, love me, to keep me safe.

When this kind of anger becomes chronic and pervasive, it leads to all kinds of health troubles. If you're an angry person, you have high-stress responses that raise your blood pressure and heart rate, increase your cholesterol, constrict your blood vessels and oxygen flow to the heart, damage your cardiovascular and immune systems, and increase your stress hormone levels, such as cortisol, which certainly cause sleep difficulties.

Psychologists claim the best way to deal with anger is to short-circuit it. It's not bad or wrong to feel anger, but left to distill in its own juices, anger soon becomes bitterness and then calcifies into resentment—that most poisonous and destructive of all emotions—and soon you have on your hands a hardened boulder of stone.

Learn to keep anger flowing by paying attention when you're angry, at what and why, so you can use anger as a liquid asset, not allowing it to harden into much more destructive emotions. Since anger flares when you're threatened and ignored, make a pact that you'll pay attention to those moments when you do get angry. Listen carefully to what your anger tells you, and then deflect it with something else.

Humor is always good; practice some relaxation exercises; breathe deeply and slowly; moan to a friend; write in your journal; exercise; pray; put things in perspective; bring some reality back into the situation; and if all else fails, just put it aside or let it go. One physical trick I've learned is to stroke the fingers of one hand over the palm of the other hand, as if stroking a lover or a small child. A feeling of safety comes over you, releasing anger and stress. Without question, holding stubbornly onto anger is something that has no place in the emotional repertoire of a dedicated sleep-seeker.

MAKE CONFESSIONS

*There is no pillow as soft as a clear
conscience.*

—FRENCH PROVERB

I KNOW MANY PEOPLE WHO LIVE THEIR LIVES dragged down by nagging, overactive, guilty consciences, shouldering shame over things they perceive they've done wrong. Perhaps this is you. You feel you're often in the wrong but feel a need to hide the fact; if anyone knew just how nasty and bad you really are, you'd live as a pariah.

This is no way to face a good, peaceful night's sleep. Confession is a tool humanity has used for millennia, and you can use it, too, to rid yourself of unnecessary guilt and clear your mind before sleep, no matter your religious preference.

Confession is a loaded word because it's linked in so many people's minds with the concepts of sin and shame. It doesn't have to be. The word *sin,* which literally means to "miss the mark," is what you believe you've done to miss doing your best; confession is owning up to it and asking to be heard and forgiven by God, yourself, your higher power, whomever you believe directs and cherishes you and the world you inhabit.

It's fairly straightforward: Once you accept the fact you're not perfect, that you make mistakes, every day—some mistakes of omission and some commission—you can spotlight your mistakes or sins, confess, and then release them. When you choose to do this during the day is up to you. Some people like to make confessions early in the morning during a prayer or meditation time. I like to review the day when I'm about to fall asleep and think of the day's events and where I could have done something better. Sometimes I know what I did was completely wrong, so that makes it easy.

Other times, it's a happenstance, where I know a different reaction would have been better—less angry, less inflexible, less over-reactive. This allows me to clear the decks, so to speak, and leave one more stress-crucible in the past, where it belongs, and not carry it into my sleep nor into my next day.

Here is an easy confession routine to start with: During your quiet time, before you fall asleep, mentally review the day, taking care to do this in a simple manner, not ruminating and restressing yourself. Pick one or two times during the day when you feel you were in the wrong or did wrong or could have simply reacted better and with more kindness. Focus on those.

Either speak them out loud to your partner (which takes courage and intimacy but nets high dividends) or mentally confess them, asking for forgiveness and, most important, help to hit the mark next time. To end your confession, give thanks for this soul-clearing opportunity.

Although you don't need a choir singing you your sins every night, it is a good idea to stay conscious of where you're off-base and where growth is possible. Resist the temptation to play either the all-good or all-bad role in any situation; try to make confessions as pragmatic and straightforward as possible. Soon you'll learn to see your unique off-the-mark paw print clearly, name and confess it, and then let it go. And you'll fall into slumber breathing much freer.

MEDITATE

Sleep is the best meditation.
−THE DALAI LAMA

THERE IS NOTHING MYSTERIOUS ABOUT MEDITA-tion. Nearly every religious tradition believes in the holding of silence as a means for spiritual growth, the East being the leader in this irenic proposal to find one's center through resting in silence. We in the West are catching up, none too early.

Many people believe that in order to practice the art, they need to become some sort of spiritual entity in saffron robe and shaved head, holding an empty golden bowl. It's a lovely image but inaccurate. Anyone with breath and the desire to unearth what's underneath all the crucial daily chit-chat can learn to meditate and reap showers of benefits spread through every part of life, sleep included.

What does meditation do? It wakes you up to a deep, sa-cred space of emptiness, where the real self dwells. All the debris—the fears and untruths—that have seeped into your body and subconscious mind are healed. In many ways it's like taking a vise off your head and heart.

If all this sounds too spiritual, suffice it to say that culti-vating inner silence and reflection brings you a deeper relax-ation than all the things you gravitate toward that keep you looking outward. Guaranteed, it will benefit your sleep.

The practical steps? You need a quiet space with phones turned off. Keep extraneous noise to a minimum. Sit on the floor on a pillow (firm meditation pillows are best) or in a straight-back chair so your spine is held taut. Place your hands gently on your knees or legs; experiment to find your best posture.

Take several very deep cleansing breaths; speak a sacred word or mantra (usually a calming one- or two-syllable word); place the word gently onto your consciousness, as if placing it on a feather, and just continue to breathe. Concentrating on the breath is what meditation is. When your mind bombards you with words and images, which it will, remain detached, and simply once again place the sacred word back lightly on the feather. Cling to nothing. Just breathe.

Two 20-minute periods, one in the morning and one in the evening, are usually recommended. If you can get only one period in, even 10 minutes, that's good to start. And if the only 10 minutes you can find are when you're lying awake in the middle of the night, try breathing and clearing your mind then. Just for practice. You may fall asleep in seconds.

UNDERSTAND YOUR NIGHTMARES

❧

*Dreaming permits each and every one
of us to be quietly and safely insane
every night of our lives.*

—DR. WILLIAM DEMENT

MANY RESTLESS SLEEPERS HAVE HIGHLY active dream lives. Nightmares are great psychic teachers but also big obstacles to restful sleep. I know, nightmares and vivid dreams were a mainstay during the fifteen years I wrestled with sound sleep. I've been labeled "Queen of the Nightmares" by more than one doctor, and if I've overcome, anyone can.

The first thing to remember: nightmares and persistent kooky dreams are not your enemies but your friends. They teach you things you'd never otherwise know if you learn to listen with an open mind. If you tune in to this "sad, healing news" (said Edgar Allen Poe, whose many story plots were known to arrive via nightmares), your subconscious mind's innate wisdom knows just what and how to tell you, how much to say, and, if you're paying attention, when to say it. It's your choice whether you want to do some work and listen or not. Understanding your disturbing dreams is work, but it pays a high dividend.

It's also helpful to realize, say sleep researchers, that what you call a nightmare may or may not actually be one. You probably think any bad dream you have during sleep is a nightmare. However, according to sleep doctors, there are four distinguishable types of nightmares occurring during different stages of sleep. (You do dream during all stages of sleep, though mostly during REM.)

1. To sleep researchers, your bad dream is an actual nightmare if it arouses you from REM sleep. You usually remember the dream, quite vividly, and although you're scared, your body usually does not react with sweating, increased pulse, and hyper-breathing. It just feels like you've been run over by a truck.

   These nightmares are generally psychological in nature, and if dream-work and journaling do not help alleviate them, psychotherapy or hypnosis often will. Once the underlying issues are resolved, the night-mares usually disappear. Sometimes, though, night-mares are like ancient agitations, strange relics that get stuck in your subconscious mind's wheel. They continue even though the causal issues clearly have been fixed. These are "bad-habit" nightmares, and you can work with these the same ways.

2. Sleep terrors, on the other hand, occur during delta, or slow-wave, sleep. This is the deepest sleep stage and is extremely hard to wake from fully. Here, the brain is half-asleep/half-awake, and terrors normally happen early at night, when delta sleep is most prevalent. In these, your body reacts: screaming, heart pounding, shivering, sweating. Yet if you turn over and go back to sleep, you'll likely not even remember this dream.

3. Often called a nightmare, isolated sleep paralysis is not considered a sleep disorder (as when it occurs with narcolepsy) but rather an extremely disconcerting intrusion of the *atonia,* or paralysis, of REM sleep carried over into your waking state. Here, your mind literally wakes up before your body, and you hear and see what's going on around you but are paralyzed.

    Many cultures call it demons-on-the-chest, and that's just what it feels like. I suffered from this type of parsimonia all through my teenage and college years. It's now suggested as a remedy that you move and circle your eyes and take deep breaths, if you can, and/or have a partner touch your body or rub and move your hands or arms or simply call your name out loud.

4. Sleep-related panic attacks that occur during stage 2 or stage 3 sleep are sometimes thought of as nightmares. They generally occur in women with daytime panic attacks. These sleep-time panics cause breathing difficulties, sweating, fear of dying or going insane, and a racing heart, just like their daytime counterparts, and are normally treated with the same medication and therapies prescribed for daytime panic attacks.

Flashbacks and anxiety attacks that appear early in the sleep cycle—at that transition between waking and sleeping (in stage 1 or in early stage 2)—are one hallmark of posttraumatic stress disorder (PTSD). Severe traumas, such as rape, physical and/or childhood sexual abuse, earthquake, war, natural disasters, extreme grief reactions, and so on, can cause this disorder. In it, you chronically "relive" the trauma(s). Treatment from a mental health professional who specializes in PTSD is best.

Many medications can and will affect both the content and quality of your dreams. Many SSRIs (selected serotonin re-uptake inhibitors used to treat depression, such as Prozac) list nightmares and/or bizarre dreams as a common (sometimes number one or two) side effect. Again, go back to the pharmaceutical pamphlet that comes with your medication or to the *Physician's Desk Reference* (PDR). Check to see if your medication is causing the vivid emotional eruptions in your dreams; it doesn't stop the pattern, but at least you know it's not your fraying soul.

Since nightmares can be as frustrating as insomnia, learning to relax is important. A doctor once told me to address my subconscious kindly a moment before I fell asleep: "My dear sweet subconscious mind (that took a while to say with sincerity), be assured I will hear what you have to tell me tonight. I can listen best if you don't shout or scare me." And, yes, this accepting attitude did work wonders for me, and still does. Once again: Dreams are only messengers. You can choose to listen or not. It's up to you.

~ NIGHTMARES ~

Our dreams are most peculiarly independent
of our consciousness and exceedingly
valuable because they cannot cheat.
—CARL JUNG

These are three nightmare-reduction suggestions that
have worked for me.

1. The brilliant twelfth-century mystic nun, Hildegard of
   Bingen, wrote in her medical work, *Liber Compositae
   Medicinae,* if you're troubled by nightmares, take one-half
   pound of betony leaves (you can find these at a Chinese
   herbalist) and wrap them in an airy piece of cloth—a nylon
   stocking will do. Stuff the herb-stocking into a lacy, airy
   pillow and place it by your face during sleep. She claims
   the "demons will fly away." Who knows? But it does
   seem to help reduce the vividness of the dreams.

2. Taking 500 mg of vitamin B1 at bedtime seems to reduce
   nightmarish dream quality, particularly during female
   PMS cycles.

3. In a journal, I write immediately upon awakening a quick
   plotline of my nightmare, along with colors, words and
   phrases, oddities, anything I can remember, and then date
   it. I make it as complete as possible and then leave it
   alone, not pondering its meaning. Usually, throughout the
   day or even the week, its message appears. I've noticed
   too much concentration makes correct interpretations flee.

LAUGH

At the far reaches of insight, wisdom
may not be far from corniness.
—STEPHEN DUNN

INSOMNIA HAS A WAY OF DRAINING JOY OUT OF life. You may think, Who can have a sense of humor on four hours of sleep? Yet laughter as the best medicine is no joke. If you're a skilled laugher, you know this already, and although it may not obliterate all your sleep struggles, it's a sure bet it'll help with other portions of your life.

In fact, studies *have* shown a correlation between laughter and lowered pulse rate, blood pressure, increased endorphins—all those sleep-enhancing goodies you seek during relaxation responses. And if you learn to regularly laugh at yourself—and at the world's conspiracies—you'll earn yourself many more friends than with a pompous, self-circled, victim attitude.

Think about it, and if you can't remember the last time you laughed, I mean really laughed hard, make a concerted effort to lighten up and start seeing what a joke life can be. Being born with a wry sense of humor helps, of course, but even comics often have trouble laughing away from the stage. There's really nothing more cathartic than hard-core laughter. (And while a wry and ironic impromptu sense of humor is the current fashion, skill as a good old-fashioned, well-rehearsed joke-teller never goes out of style.)

Years ago, I interviewed the late Norman Cousins, in what unfortunately turned out to be one of the last interviews he gave. A very pragmatic allopath (one who practices Western medicine), Dr. Cousins nonetheless detailed in his many books his firm belief that he cured himself of serious illness through daily laughter.

Though our interview was serious (the topic was AIDS), I knew better than to leave without asking whether he thought daily prompted laughter could help insomnia. "My dear girl," he chuckled, "I think it's the *only* thing that can cure it."

SKYWATCH AND BE MINDFUL

*Late on the third day, at the
very moment when, at sunset, we were
making our way through a herd of
hippopotamuses, there flashed upon
my mind, unforeseen and unsought,
the phrase, "Reverence for life."*

—ALBERT SCHWEITZER

DO YOU KNOW WHAT THE CLOUDS LOOKED like today? Here in Los Angeles County at dusk, a long sheet of cirrus clouds streaked down the center of a mulberry-lit sky. Gorgeous. As I walked this evening, I watched and did not see one person look or glance up at the sky.

We live in a stunning world, and what a shame to flash by it on a regular basis. Three things on this planet anchor us to the fact that we're basically wind-swept flecks in an unhurried cosmos: the ocean, the mountains, and the celestial patterns in the sky.

While not everyone is lucky enough to have a view of the mountains or the sea, everyone gets an equal opportunity look at the sky, 24/7, for free. If you were one of those kids who loved to lie on your back and stare for hours at the clouds making strange shapes, try to revive some of that youngster. It will help your mind learn a relaxing technique, *mindful attention,* and is a de-stressor par excellence.

Being mindful, or practicing "mindfulness," is really nothing more than paying attention to where you are paying attention. If your attention is spread thin and not focused on something immediate, you dilute the one true thing you have in your possession, this second. Learning how to focus on the present instead of somewhere else minimizes anxiety and stress, two notorious sleep-stealers.

So whether you're eating breakfast, taking a shower, or looking at the Italian night sky, in mindful practice, your mind is on what's happening now, not something else. It's your choice, of course, but be mindful, at least, that you're choosing not to be mindful.

Some cultures are better than others at holding up mindful attention as something golden. A competitive culture, like ours, almost by definition would need to bill forward/future thinking as important. Unfortunately, for most people over the age of ten, skywatching would probably fall under the "Do something constructive!" category.

Small but important things, like taking note of the sky every day, help you learn more mindful habits, which then naturally spill over into other areas of your life. A lovely and easy exercise is to jot down the sky's cloud formations for a week or two or more in your journal. You'll soon see that no matter whether you have a good night's sleep or not, the clouds will still be swirling, never to look the same again. Which, in paradox, only improves your sleep.

CRY AT NIGHT IF YOU WANT TO

I fell into such a weeping, it wept me. . . .
—HEATHER MCHUGH

I F THERE'S SOME THING YOUR BED IS FOR, IT'S rest and release and rejuvenation and self-expression— be it sleep, sex, dreaming, honest pillow breath-talks, or crying. I find that tucked in bed, deeply relaxed, this is a captive place to release feelings and cry.

If you're alone, of course, this will be easier to do than if you're with a partner, but crying late at night—or crying yourself to sleep, as it were—is not something negative. Rather, it is highly releasing and positive. Crying *is* cathartic.

I'm always stunned by the number of friends who can't remember the last time they cried. If I had to count this figure, my abacus would have broken long ago, quite possibly never to be repaired. If you have a concern about your image, remember your bed is the most intimate place you inhabit. Where else to better let your guard drop and your feelings simmer and seep out?

In this postpsychoanalytic age, crying is sanctioned as therapeutic and a good form of immediate pain relief. Still, my guess is many men, and some women, would see this as dependent and silly: Why cry if you're not in real pain? Women are blessed, thank goodness, as tears are a much more natural part of our lives. Every woman knows a good cry is as good as swimming through sweet syrup.

There have been times I've been perfectly happy, in fact, had a good day, and I'll still crawl in bed and sob. This might sound weird to some, but what if I stuffed those feelings in—would it not disturb my sleep? Or worse, my health? What are tears for except for release and healing? Often they don't have anything to do with the day but rather with much deeper feelings, of past unresolved griefs, hurts, angers, and fears.

What I think happens when you allow yourself to cry at night is that you release the subconscious mind and let it know you're willing to listen. You won't be fighting it. Let it come and tell you what you need to know while you sleep, and be grateful for both dreams and tears. And do remember: It's your bed and it's your party and you can cry if you want to.

BLESS AND BE GRATEFUL

*Now blessings light on him that
first invented this same sleep. It covers
a man all over, thoughts and all,
like a cloak.*

—CERVANTES, *DON QUIXOTE*

GRATITUDE IS AN ELIXIR, CHANGING THE LIFE of the grateful like nothing else. It's a fashionable topic, now, how to become more grateful, but not particularly a difficult thing to master. In essence, you just need to wake up, stay awake, and comment thankfully on what you see. And always be mindful that a chronic, ungrateful attitude is a high-risk activity.

There are many ways to practice gratitude in your life. You can use your journal, once again, or a separate notepad, and jot down daily one or two things you appreciated most during the past 24 hours. For those who have sleep difficulties, doing this at night, just before retiring, is best. It brings a sense of calm to the subconscious mind, like planting a seed of positive sunlight in your brain, letting it gradually heal your subconscious wounds.

Of course, it's important to give genuine thanks for those blessings; you didn't earn them, they are gifts. Sincerity is an obvious requirement. When I first started out, I used to think of them as daily thank you notes, which I'd never forget to send a friend. Why ignore the Creator?

Today, I use a Jesuit practice, *examen*. In it, I routinely go over the one moment for which I am most grateful and that most connected me to God and life; and then I name the one moment for which I am least grateful or that made me feel least connected to God and life. Done faithfully at night, this practice has helped millions of people since Saint Ignatius of Loyola's time to locate what fosters and what doesn't foster love, life, blessing—and gratitude—in your life.

A story about World War II refugee children in the book *Sleeping with Bread: Holding What Gives You Life* explains how a group of youngsters could not fall asleep at night, so burdened were they from past traumas. They were terrified that somehow the next day they'd wake up to again having no food or shelter. It was a sleepless little lot until someone came upon the clever idea of having the children each hold a piece of bread during the night, which allowed them to fall readily asleep.

It's a great story about the power of planting in your mind at bedtime that simple seed of gratitude and security, letting it permeate your subconscious. With daily gratitude practice, that great stressmonger, fear—about being safe, having enough, being loved—dissipates as you recognize that your blessings aren't going to disappear, that instead they arrive daily. Hoarding and envy dissolve, and you can truly relax. A much, much better frame of mind with which to fall asleep.

CHAPTER 7

SLEEP HAZARDS

DO NOT EAT LATE AT NIGHT

❧

Life itself is the proper binge.
–JULIA CHILD

LISTEN, THERE'S JUST ABOUT NOTHING BETTER than a late-night snack—cereal, sandwich, the cold glutonosity of ice cream, whatever. That's on the emotional side. Physically, it's about the worst thing you can do if you want to help relax your body and prepare it for sleep. Your digestive system will have to spend its precious energy during the night digesting this food instead of resting and repairing. That's something you want to avoid at all costs.

The rule to remember about food and the pleasure of eating: When you rest, all of you should rest—including your stomach.

To do this, simply avoid heavy meals within 4 or 5 hours of bedtime. Try to keep to this rule as much as possible. It may be hard with today's schedules, but if your bedtime is at 10 P.M., that means dinner should be around 6 P.M. How many people do you know who get home late, eat heavily at 8 P.M., and then fall asleep at 10 P.M.? This is not sound physiological science. Get into a routine of eating late—particularly the midnight snack—and without question, you're asking for sleep trouble.

If you can, make your last dinner meal the lightest meal of the day, an inversion of the pre–health food days when coffee and cigarettes were breakfast, a near-nothing was lunch, and a lacuna meal sufficed at night. It's much better to have a solid breakfast with plenty of protein and then graze through the day, eating five or six smaller, lighter meals. Think of yourself as an engine that burns fuel much more efficiently when it is pumped in at regular intervals.

It's also true that if you are starved, dieting, or just plain hungry, your sleep will likewise be affected, with a possible drop in blood sugar, so you awaken during the night. To avoid this possibility, a late-night, light-carbohydrate snack, say, a banana or apple, with a little bit of protein, such as a small piece of cheese or a soy protein drink, can help stave off rumblings while also raising serotonin levels and helping you stay asleep. You should have the snack about 1 to 2 hours before bedtime, though some people eat it right before falling asleep. See what works best for your system.

Anything with the amino acid tryptophan (bananas, cheese, milk, yogurt, turkey, dates, figs), which converts in the brain to serotonin and helps modulate sleep (the process takes 45 minutes to an hour), eases you into slumber. Also, the proverbial warm glass of milk an hour or so before bed helps improve sleep onset and deepen sleep. Try it with a touch of honey and nutmeg or, like the British, cowslips.

Here's a drink I often use about an hour before bed for prebedtime stomach grumblings: Mix soy protein powder, almond milk, a banana for tryptophan, and a touch of nutmeg for spice. Resist any subterranean outlaw streak that urges you to dump in any other foods with fat, sugar, or caffeine. Stop rubbing shoulders with the midnight munchies; it's a guaranteed quick sleep-enhancer.

CHECK YOUR VITAMINS
AND MINERALS

❧

The average, healthy, well-adjusted
adult gets up at seven-thirty in the
morning feeling just plain terrible.

—JEAN KERR

I F YOU THINK THE WHOLE VITAMIN/MINERAL/
health food craze is nothing but a modern version of
medicinal snake oil, this section isn't for you. However,
if you see the vital link among vitamins, minerals, what you
eat, and your sleep patterns, read on. These life building
blocks are great soporifics and help adjust sleep patterns if
you hit the right levels and combinations for your body. This
is one arena in which a serious chunk of my own insomnia
was knocked off its pedestal.

Following is a discussion of major nutrients your body
needs for restful sleep. Check off ones you think you may
need, and then discuss them with your doctor, nutritionist,
or other health professional.

Something to remember: Megadoses of anything can be
harmful, and the wrong extra nutrients for your body can
do more harm than good. While all bodies need certain levels of vitamins and minerals for optimum health and well-
being, women need variations of many levels and often
either don't know or don't have enough time to correct the

situation. However, it's an equation well worth the time and effort to set up correctly, and a big benefactor is your sleep.

Without question, the best source of nutrients is from fresh food itself. Yet with depleted soil, pesticides, processed foods, and our bad but prolific habit of eating food too quickly, assimilating the proper amounts of nutrients from food is difficult. A multiple vitamin and mineral tablet or capsule is the best start. Then see if you need "boosters" in any of the following areas, taking into account the two total amounts—from both your multivitamin and your supplement.

Calcium and magnesium deficiencies are two major culprits of disturbed sleep among women. Calcium is one of the most abundant minerals in the body and yet something most women still need fortified. All women need extra calcium (1,200 mg premenopause and 1,500 mg post-menopause), particularly as we age. Calcium has a calming effect on the nervous system, helps promote restful and high quality sleep, and is good to take right at bedtime. It's also important, of course, for strong bones and staving off osteo-porosis. Calcium citrate and calcium carbonate have the edge for best absorption. Some good sources for calcium: dairy products, soy milk, nuts (especially almonds), onions, tanger-ines, and lemons.

Magnesium also has a calming effect on the brain and nervous system and is important for good sleep. It's a natural sedative and helps the body absorb calcium and is often combined with calcium in tablet form. A suggested daily magnesium intake is 300 mg to 500 mg. It's found in plenty of foods: dark green vegetables, seafood, whole grains, nuts, seeds, dairy foods, legumes, and fruits.

Insufficient copper and iron levels can also cause poor sleep. Copper is involved in making norepinephrine, a brain chemical responsible for the brain's general arousal and crucially involved in sleep; and iron is essential for making dopamine, also involved in sleep. Since too much copper and iron can cause serious side effects, take these supplements only under the guidance of a nutritionist or health professional. Good sources: eggs, nuts, seafood, and molasses.

The B-vitamins regulate the body's use of tryptophan and other amino acids and are depleted by stress, birth control pills, smoking, and alcohol. Most all B-vitamins are important in maintaining good sleep and general well-being. Start with a complete B-complex and then experiment with some of the following single Bs for boosters: niacin (B3), pantothenic acid (B5), pyridoxine (B6), folic acid (B9); choline and inosital are all important B-vitamins for sleep (check with a professional for dosage). Vitamin B12 can also help, particularly if you're a vegetarian.

Make sure you are taking enough vitamins A, D (important for sunlight synthesis and calcium absorption), C (important for stressed adrenals), and E (as an anti-oxidant), especially during winter months when sunlight is reduced.

If you think your multivitamin isn't giving you enough dosage, consult your health-care professional and work out a supplement plan that's not too overwhelming. Ingesting too many tablets is taxing and daunting unless you're fully committed. Be assured, though, you'll feel a difference in your sleep if you give it time.

SKIP THE NAPS

*There is no point at which you can say,
well, I'm successful now. I might as
well take a nap.*

—CARRIE FISHER

FOR THE CHRONICALLY FATIGUED, THIS SEEMS somewhat Stalinistic: No afternoon naps. Naps, after all, are not only one of life's great little pleasures but are also making a resounding comeback in popular society. Books, magazine articles, medical health advice, and Web sites all suggest the afternoon nap as a way to recharge depleted batteries in a hyper world.

Maybe so. Yet for those who struggle with fitful nighttime sleep, naps are off limits. Why? It's not hard to figure out. Sleeping 2 or more hours in the afternoon will obviously effect your nighttime sleep patterns. After a long nap, you're not as tired, you stay up later, your mind is rested and more alert, but unfortunately your deepest sleep has already been spent. No matter how you stack it, if you're a poor sleeper—and until you become a steadily good one—forget naps.

However, there is a sweet caveat. According to some sleep experts, the "power nap"—a short, crunched mid-afternoon nap—is in. This is a nap not like the juicy 2 to 3 hour snooze, but a crisp nap anywhere from 10 to no more than 40 to 45 minutes. Time here is the essential element. (You can think of Salvador Dali, who sat in a chair holding a spoon with a tin plate underneath, and when he fell asleep and the spoon dropped, he awoke finished and refreshed, nap over.)

The power nap—and, again, if you fall in the insomniac category, it's the only one you should try at this point—must be kept short. Less than 30 minutes is best, but many people who nap for only 10 to 15 minutes claim they feel fabulous. The shorter the nap, the less likely your brain will tumble into your nighttime sleep pattern, causing you to wake up with sleep inertia, that groggy, disoriented, spacey haze.

You'll want to make sure your nap goes well, so if you're self-employed, you've got the home advantage. If you work in an outside office, you'll need a few extra steps. For work-time naps, plan and announce your naps to yourself and colleagues and get your napping materials together (store a favorite blanket or pillow in your desk or closet).

At work, set aside times for regular naps with phones turned off, calls held, beepers off. A "Do Not Disturb" sign would be appropriate here. Set your alarm clock, let your mind drift off, and simply float downstream. If you're at home during the day, it's easy. Again, turn off the phones, shut the door, set the alarm, and fall on to your bed. Make sure you set regularized daily nap times, at least as close as possible.

The best time to nap is during the daily afternoon energy lull, from 1 P.M. to 3 P.M., no later than 4 P.M. This is the circadian rhythm's natural dip, when body temperature drops slightly almost exactly 12 hours after your strongest nighttime pressure to fall asleep, around 1 A.M. to 3 A.M. It seems nature was on our side all along, building in nap time, which, by the way, is just about everyone's favorite memory of kindergarten.

If you're pregnant, a brand new mother, sick, grieving, under extreme emotional and/or physical stress, your body does need the extra sleep. But if you notice your naps are causing fitful nighttime sleep—ease off. Waking up refreshed in the morning is the most important thing.

AVOID CAFFEINE, NICOTINE, SUGAR, AND ALCOHOL

*Eliminate something superfluous from
your life. Break a habit. Do something
that makes you feel insecure.*

—PIERO FERNICCI

B Y NOW I'M SURE YOU KNOW ALL ABOUT THE evils of caffeine, nicotine, alcohol, carbonated drinks, and sugar, and how they all affect your body. Well, they affect your sleep patterns, too.

Despite whatever else is going on in your life and whatever else may or may not contribute to your sleep difficulties, if you want to be sure to have a lousy night's sleep, smoke, drink plenty of caffeinated coffee and tea, some alcohol, gulp down lots of soft drinks, and eat good, gooey, sugar stuff all day long.

If you want to sleep better and in general feel better and be healthier, don't do any of those things. There's really not much else to say about abstaining from things like caffeine (the most widely used psychoactive drug in the world) and nicotine (second most widely used legal drug) and sugar (America's number one dietary addiction) except that it's a tough discipline—at first. But once your body gets used to the removal of poisons from its system, it becomes quite easy. Believe it or not.

Still, it amazes me how many people, knowing all the health hazards of such poor eating and health habits, indulge daily, thinking somehow the chemicals they ingest are different when they enter *their* bodies. It's said Americans drink 400 million cups of coffee daily, second only to water. Caffeine, which, in coffee, comes from the same plant as cocaine, works by binding to bodily receptors and stimulating synapse contractions. Less fatigue and the lift.

Yet consuming more than 200 mg of caffeine a day (which is only about two cups of coffee, two or three cola drinks, several ounces of chocolate, or several caffeine-containing pain capsules) is said to affect sleep and create caffeine addiction. It also takes about 3 to 7 hours to rid your system completely of caffeine, depending on age and metabolism. That's not a whole lot of intake.

And while everyone's body reacts differently to caffeine and how it's metabolized, studies show that insomniacs generally are more aroused and metabolically stimulated anyhow, even without caffeine. As you age, your body also metabolizes caffeine more slowly. If you can't go cold turkey on caffeine and think you still want some in your diet, try to limit your intake to under 200 mg and before noontime. This way there is much less chance of disturbed sleep.

Nicotine, on the other hand, is an even more powerful stimulant than caffeine and obviously much more dangerous to your health. Eliminate it. Studies are conclusive that smokers have more difficulty falling asleep because cigarettes raise blood pressure and heart rate and stimulate brainwave activity. And though I've never smoked enough to become addicted—only minorly in college—I do know the power of this addiction and how stressful it is to quit.

Yet studies show clearly that even with the horrors of nicotine withdrawal, you'll sleep much better almost straightaway after only a few weeks. You'll likely fall asleep faster and wake less during the night and, goodness knows, won't be lighting up and stimulating yourself even more when you wake up and try to relax at 3 A.M.

And about that nightcap doctors used to prescribe: yes, alcohol will make you initially more sleepy and may help you fall asleep faster, but its soporific benefits last only during the first half of the night, when you have a lot of slow-wave deep sleep but with your REM dreaming periods sharply reduced. The second half of the night, you'll wake more often and have much poorer and more fragmented sleep, often with REM intruding upon other sleep stages, depriving your body of deep rest.

Sugar is also a large sleep-robber, and ingesting too much (particularly late at night) throws your blood sugar off, possibly causing blood sugar drops in the middle of the night. Not only will ridding your system of too much sugar maintain healthy weight and better health in general, but it will also help with healthy sleep.

Try to give up just one of these system poisons, and do it cold turkey if you can (always consult your doctor first); go for one or two months or so and then go cold turkey on another one (again, check with your physician). Tackle them like you would debt on credit cards—one at a time, keep at it, and soon you'll be free.

BEWARE OF SLEEPING PILLS

*My sleeping capsule, my red
and blue zeppelin, drops me from a
terrible altitude.*

—SYLVIA PLATH

NO ONE CAN TELL YOU NOT TO TAKE A SLEEP-
ing pill. In fact, sleeping pills do work. Serious side
effects, however, make them less than a prime
choice, and education is important if you choose to follow
this route. Often, sleeping pills (or hypnotics) are the one re-
liable tool allopathic physicians have in their arsenal, and
they often reach for their prescription pad out of mere lack
of alternatives. You will, therefore, need to be a well-informed patient.

In the early 1960s, the Benzodiazepine (BZs) group of
drugs appeared on the medical scene and are today still the
preferred allopathic drug for treating insomnia. During the
1970s, these sleeping pills were the most widely prescribed
medications in the world, and despite reduced usage, they
still represent big business for pharmaceutical companies,
accounting for approximately $400 million in annual sales.

How do they work? BZs promote sleep by depressing the
brain's activity and slowing brain waves. They're believed to
reduce the time required to fall asleep, decrease the number
and duration of nighttime awakenings, and increase total

sleep time. Although all BZs are about equal in effectiveness in inducing sleep, they do differ in terms of their half-life (the time it takes for the body to break down and eliminate half of the drug taken). This affects next-day drowsiness, or "hangover," a common complaint with sleeping pill medication. The newer Ambien and Sonata have relatively short half-lives.

Here are the most prescribed BZs, both their brand and generic names:

Ambien (zolpidem)
Ativan (lorazepam)
Dalmane (flurazepam)
Doral (quazepam)
Halcion (triazolam)
Klonopin (clonazepam)
Prosom (estazolam)
Restoril (Temazepam)
Serax (oxazepam)
Sonata (zaleplon)
Tranxene (clorazepate)
Valium (diazepam)
Xanax (alprazolam)

What's the problem with taking sleeping pills? There are many, but mainly, although they may be moderately effective in the short term, sooner or later all lose their effectiveness. This is because, with continued use, the brain gets accustomed, or "habituated," to their effects. Physicians are advised not to prescribe BZs for more than a two- to three-week period at a time, some for four to six weeks maximum. (How many people do you know who take these drugs for years?)

BZs lessen deep sleep and REM sleep and increase stage 2 sleep, the one semispurious sleep stage. They cut down on stages 3 and 4 (the most restorative stages), so sleep is of a poorer quality. They also can produce hangover effects and "rebound" insomnia—a more intense insomnia than originally experienced, which occurs when people attempt to halt their usage.

If the drugs are taken long enough, physical dependency occurs, and classic withdrawal symptoms such as anxiety, headaches, nausea, and even seizures can appear, particularly if the drugs are stopped cold turkey. Tolerance dependence is another problem, so you'll gradually need increasing dosages for the drug to work. If you do become dependent, you will need to work out a reduction schedule with your doctor; don't try to go it alone.

Bottom line: Sleeping pills are a short-term method for people with transient insomnia. Most insomniacs have broader issues and do well to investigate other methods of treatment, ones that attempt not merely to alleviate symptoms of disturbed sleep disorder but to also dig down to the root causes we so dearly want to get at. I'm sure you know as many people as I do who regularly recount their sad sleeping-pill horror stories. Once inside, it can be a labyrinth to navigate.

It's not a sin, and the search for a holy grail sleep aid is hardly a new one. Be informed, and consider your alternatives carefully before you gulp.

UNDERSTAND FOOD ALLERGIES

*Does the cosmic space we
dissolve into taste of us then?*
—RAINER MARIA RILKE

HIDDEN FOOD ALLERGIES CAN AFFECT YOUR sleep just like any other allergy can. Many of us seemingly sail through life not aware—or perhaps not fully intending to find out—what foods trigger minor allergic reactions in our bodies.

Strictly speaking, food allergies are not the same thing as food intolerances: food allergies are the body's immune response to a specific food and involve the release of histamine into the bloodstream. If it's a severe reaction, it can lead to a life-threatening situation—anaphylactic shock.

Food intolerances, on the other hand, do not involve the immune system and the release of histamine. Food intolerances sometimes provoke similar reactions, though, like hives, swelling, itching, or can have little symptomology at all. However, for language purposes, food allergy and food intolerances are used to cover the broad spectrum.

Since allergies arise from at least two main sources—hereditary weakness and overuse or abuse of a generally harmless food or substance—you have some potential information right up front. If your entire family is allergic to milk products, it's a good guess you might be, too. Yet it's the latter—abused substances—that are easier to identify. And once you know what food is causing you difficulty, wisdom suggests you remove it from your diet, or at least drastically reduce it.

Perhaps you've heard that food allergy testing is an expensive and tedious procedure, which it admittedly is if you choose to follow only the traditional medical route. What follows is the best and easiest way I learned to narrow the search-and-find food allergy trap before you move on to more expensive medical testing. (Consult a nutritionist and/or your physician to gain further help in determining your unique food allergens. They can help you determine if you need to see an allergy specialist for definite medical analysis.)

Make a long and very complete list of all the foods and drinks you regularly consume. Do this through use of a daily log for several weeks, or you can trust your memory, as long as you're accurate. Be sure to include substances like gum, tobacco, alcohol, carbonated drinks, tea, coffee, dessert, even breath mints, or everything you regularly stick in your mouth.

Divide the foods and various substances into four categories: (1) *Must have* foods, (2) *Favorite* foods, (3) *OK* foods, (4) *Infrequent* foods, listing them according to preference. (Make your number one selections those that are your favorite foods and substances—ones you feel you can't do well without and would be hard to stop—and move on down the list until you've covered your complete diet.)

An odd biological law says that you tend to become most easily addicted to those things that are the worst for you, for example, sugar, tobacco, alcohol, drugs. Addiction and allergies often go hand in glove. Hence, the foods in your highest categories—the ones you eat the most—are the ones to which you may be most allergic. If you have a chocolate frozen yogurt daily in the afternoon or eggs each morning and love them, they're probably number one on your list.

Once identified, avoid as many of your number one foods and drinks as possible for one month or so. If your health and sleep seem improved, you've found some allergens you can then either choose to live with or without.

Here's a short list of some of the most common food allergens today:

Chocolate
Coffee and caffeinated drinks
Corn
Dairy products
Eggs
Food additives
Peanuts
Seafood
Sugar
Tobacco
Wheat
Yeast

You may think there's nothing else to consume, but, ah, there is. And if your sleep improves, you now have a new dietary, sleep-enhancing plan.

TAKE YOUR MEDICATIONS, BUT...

❧

I am slippery, I am slipping, two weeks
now without my medication.
—LAUREN SLATER

IF YOU HAVE A CHRONIC ILLNESS THAT REQUIRES long-term medication—such as heart disease, asthma, depression or mood disorder, Multiple Sclerosis, HIV, migraines, or any of the auto-immune disorders, the list goes on—you'll likely ingest potent (and helpful and needed) medications for a long period of time. However, there are side effects. Period. There's no way around this fact.

Your body thus needs extra help to detoxify and clean out your system, something frequently overlooked by allo-pathic-trained medical professionals. Until they do some catching up (which won't benefit you now), this is your job.

Cleaning out your body and internal organs so they operate at optimal levels will take much time, experimentation, effort, money, commitment, and discipline. And lots of persistence and patience. However, I would go so far as to say anyone who has to take long-term or lifetime medications needs to commit with the same concern they give all their other health needs, to giving their body and organs the optimal clean environment with which to do their job.

If you smoke, drink alcohol, use recreational drugs, live in a particularly polluted environment, eat a high-fat, sugary, fast-food diet—or you did any of these things for an extended period in your past—you'll be that much more behind the scrimmage line. (Please see chapter 5 for internal detoxification and cleansing suggestions.)

Not only will chronic medications cause internal pollution, as it were, but certain medications also strongly effect sleep patterns. Don't ignore this. Check your medications and see if what you take has any potential insomniac side effects.

You want to not only speak with your doctor about your medication's side effects but also do some research on your own. Ask your pharmacist for the medication insert printed by the company and sold with the original bottle. It will list all side effects, even slight ones: your doctor may not be familiar with the less egregious ones.

Look up your medications and their side effects in the *Physician's Desk Reference;* get on the Internet and do some more research. If you still think your medication is affecting your sleep and if all else fails, call the company and speak to someone in product development or to the company's staff pharmacist—something I have done when at my wits' end.

Sometimes you just know what you know, and though the printout might not list insomnia as a side effect, it may interact with your particular chemistry that way. My attitude: If companies make billions of dollars from a product, they can listen to and help one of their customers who has a sleep complaint.

Medications that can cause sleep difficulties and insomnia are too prolific to list here, so if you're taking any medications, the first step is to find out if the medication is a culprit. If it is, then you and your doctor can best discuss your next step.

SILENCE SNORING SPOUSES

❧

*There ain't no way to find out why a
snorer can't hear himself snore.*

—MARK TWAIN

WHETHER IT'S WINDOW-RATTLING SNORING or gasping-for-air snorts, there are things to do short of grabbing a samurai sword. (Ask sleep specialists the number one complaint at their first appointment: it's usually from a partner demanding that the #$% snoring end.) As many as 40 million Americans disruptively snore each night, so it's no small situation.

Loud snorers are an interesting lot. Since they usually don't know anything about their nighttime sawing—excessive daytime sleepiness is usually the signal for them—it rests on the partner to take control of the chaos, unless you're the rare individual who can sleep through such a symphony.

First, recognize that your partner may have a medical condition: obstructive sleep apnea (see chapter 1), in which airflow to the lungs is briefly blocked repeatedly during the night with each episode—and there can be hundreds nightly—lasting as long as a minute. Listen to the snoring: if it's soft and steady, it may mean there's some mild airway passage change. If you can deal with it, probably no need for concern.

However, if the airway is completely blocked and the snoring stops and starts with snorts or loud gasps and with clicking sounds as the airway tries to open, be concerned and push your snorer to the doctor fast. Sleep apnea can affect—as well as be a symptom of—cardiovascular health, as well as affect other health issues.

How to convince the snorer he snores and needs medical help? The sweet and gentle approach is good, but if resistance lasts longer than a couple of months and your own sleep is suffering, make a deal. Either he sees a doctor or he needs to move to another room to sleep. (Why should you give up your bed?) At some point down the not-too-long-road, he'll end up in the doctor's office (best is an ear, nose, and throat specialist), and an effective strategy can be implemented.

Until that time, try these famed antisnoring techniques:

Nudge or kick your partner so he changes positions.

Use a humidifier to help increase moisture in the room (swollen membranes from dryness can cause snoring).

Discourage your partner's nighttime alcohol and/or tranquilizer use.

Suggest he take off some pounds (be nice).

Suggest she stop smoking (less nice).

Experiment with antisnoring dental appliances.

Check for allergies, either environmental or food.

For yourself, try the new wireless headphones and use some white noise or soothing nature sounds.

Help him learn to sleep on his side.

If all else fails, you can do what a colleague of mine did: Her husband refused to believe he made a peep at night, so she taped him making his zoo sounds and played it on his voice machine every morning, so it was the first message he got at work. He finally did get the message.

HALT CALLING KIDS

Sleep, riches and health, to be truly
enjoyed, must be interrupted.
—JEAN PAUL FIEHTER

THE "SLEEPING LIKE A BABY" MISNOMER HAS fooled more than one new mother into a state of panic when her infant helps pile up her sleep debt— estimated at 500 to 750 hours the first year alone! Infants and children seem to sleep a lot, but their sleep patterns are much different from adults', which is sometimes hard to re- member in the early wee hours. Some basic information and a few tips can help ease some of the draining fatigue and nighttime chaos.

Normally, a newborn infant sleeps between 16 and 20 hours a day, but the sleep is very fragmented (not until about three months of age will an infant begin to sleep through the night—though statistics suggest 10 percent of lucky par- ents have a champion night sleeper at one month).

The baby's deep sleep is utterly deep (researchers have tried with extremely high decibels to wake infants to no avail), and their dream time, or REM sleep, is heavily skewed, with about 10 hours of REM sleep per 4 hours of wake time. (One French study found that at 25 weeks or so, the in vitro infant dreams virtually nonstop!) Remember, through all of this your baby is learning how to sleep.

You'll get a morning and afternoon nap out of a toddler until perhaps age one or two, and at about age two to six years the afternoon nap shifts out. This is where the whining and delayed bed techniques usually start to appear.

Many child sleep specialists, including Dr. Richard Ferber, who wrote the classic *Solve Your Child's Sleep Problems*, promote taking the sleep reins early in your child's life. Ferber advises parents to pick a schedule that's right for themselves and their babies and then stick to it, letting the tiny tot gradually cry or scream it out for a week or so until they learn to soothe themselves to sleep.

Here are some suggestions for sleep-deprived moms to help establish a more regular, all-night sleep pattern in their kids:

- Don't wake a sleeping baby, even for a scheduled feeding, and make sure your baby has a full feeding at day's end.
- Keep the infant's room quiet and dark at night, and during feeding or changing, limit movement, noise, talking, and other stimulation.
- Likewise, expose infants to bright light, activities, and stimulation during the day, which helps establish a consistent body-temperature rhythm.
- Infants and toddlers need a wind-down bedtime ritual just like adults. Make it consistent: read a book, sing a lullaby, or use gentle rocking, but with low lights.
- Help your infants learn to fall asleep on their own by putting them in the crib before they fall asleep.

For toddlers:

- An "attachment" or transitional object, such as a stuffed toy or blanket, helps children limit their nightly mom-awakenings.
- Make sure kids limit indoor TV watching and low physical activity and engage in outdoor movement.
- Limit consumption of caffeinated foods and beverages—caffeine has a much stronger affect on kids than on adults and disrupts sleep more.
- Keep the wind-down bedtime routine strict and stable, and keep TV out of your child's bedroom and limit late-night watching.
- If the child has nighttime fears, leave a night-light on or keep the door ajar, and limit their exposure to frightening TV or videotape images.
- Don't use early bedtime as a punishment, as this re-enforces a negative sleep stimulus.
- Don't engage in interaction when your child wakes you in the middle of the night or keeps getting up from bed; put them back in bed and tell them it's okay and that they're safe, say sweet dreams, and leave. Promoting delayed behavior only increases it (unless, of course, your child is sick or under undue stress). Then go back to sleep and hope your child does, too.

PREVENT AND OVERCOME JET LAG

❧

It is the East and Juliet is the Sun.

—WILLIAM SHAKESPEARE,
ROMEO AND JULIET

FOR THOSE WHO FREQUENTLY FLY, AND WHO also have delicate sleep cycles, jet lag is trouble. As with everything involving sleep, some people are more affected than others, but it's a pretty good guess that if you have sleep troubles at home, jet lag will only exacerbate them.

Jet lag occurs when you travel quickly across several time zones, causing your internal biological rhythm to shift out of sync with new local time. Fatigue, nonrestorative sleep, slowed reactions, and stomach and intestinal problems are just a few of jet lag's well-known symptoms.

It's usually most noticeable after crossing three or more time zones, as longer flights cause havoc with your internal rhythms more heavily. Eastbound flights shorten the day, whereas westbound flights lengthen the day. (Flying north or south causes no rhythm fluctuations.) Thus, night and day, light and dark tumble out of order.

All of the body's rhythms are affected by jet lag. Since circadian rhythms involve a number of daily physical cycles, such as hormone function and body temperature, among many others, all these have to catch up to local time, each doing so at a different rate.

Two differing schools suggest how to battle this unpleasant travel companion. One group advocates immediately resetting your sleep clock to the new destination, whereas others propose keeping your sleep and wake patterns set to your home time zone. You'll have to find which method works best for you.

To reset your clock to a new time zone: On a Los Angeles to London flight, you should not go to sleep upon arrival but immediately get out into the sunlight and then go to bed at your normal time, but on London time. Alternatively, if you follow the second group's suggestion, upon arrival go to bed straightaway if it's your bedtime, and sleep until your normal rising hour.

Either way, after a few days your body readjusts. Since light and dark primarily reset circadian rhythms, it's crucial to get into the sun either upon arrival or early the next morning if you arrive at night. The sun does the evolutionary brainwork for you. There are things, however, you can do to cut down on jet lag's effects, beginning well before you step on the aircraft.

Get a full night's sleep before the trip: jet lag's effects are much higher if you're already running a sleep debt. Try to choose a flight that follows the sun. When flying east, fly early in the day; when flying west, fly late.

Anticipate your new time zone: If you're flying when it's nighttime at your destination, try to sleep on the plane. Use a sleep mask or close the window and use a pillow. If it's daytime at your destination, stay awake.

As with all flying, drink lots of water and avoid caffeine and alcohol. Stretch and breathe and walk about the cabin as much as possible. It's important upon arrival to stay outdoors in sunlight. If you want, you can even bring a full-spectrum light to your new destination; just check voltage and outlets.

When I arrive at my new destination, I always keep an eye on my body temperature. I make the new room a little on the cool side; try to take a hot bath 2 hours before bed and warm up in the morning with a hot breakfast, exercise, or even a rising-with-the-sun walk. Avoiding my penchant for sunglasses, I always let my naked eyes have as much sunlight as possible. I try to eat light for a few days, as my daily digestive rhythm takes a while to catch up. I also rely on calming aromatherapy formulas (such as lavender and sandalwood) when sleep is desired and stimulating formulas (peppermint and eucalyptus) when I want to stay awake. Learning how to deal with jet lag assures a better night's sleep no matter where your head lays.

SLEEP STRATEGIES
FOR SHIFT WORKERS

Day or night, good sleep is your right.
−DAVID MORGAN

L ITTLE CAN DISRUPT SLEEP CYCLES MORE THAN
erratic shift work. Women seem prone to heightened
fatigue and sleepiness in shift work, even more than
men. It may have something to do with innate biological
rhythms or just the fact that women generally have more
work to do at home than men, another extra shift.

However, if you do shift work, there are some tips to help
regulate and better structure your sleep habits so you sleep
and work at peak efficiency, avoiding chronic exhaustion.

If you work in service industries such as health care, in
action 24 hours, it's likely you respond as most shift workers
do, sleeping days when on the night shift and then immediately shifting back to a day schedule when you're off. Here,
your unfortunate biological clock can't figure out what part
of the day cycle you're in. Knowledge about your body clock
and circadian rhythm is important for smooth shift worker
sleep.

Your body clock is located in the hypothalamus, deep inside your brain. This is the network that deals with fatigue,
food intake, hunger, thirst, endocrine levels, sex drive, anger,
among other things. This body clock tends to run slowly for
still unknown reasons, generally on a 25-hour cycle. This

helps shift work if your shift rotates clockwise, from day to evening to night.

Your body's clock resets itself daily, and the best resetter is the sun. Shift work inverts this important cue. Like all time-pieces, your body clock is delicate and needs to adjust to time shifts. Pulling it from day to night to evening to day shifts is a sure way to wreak sleep havoc.

Here are some tips to alleviate potential shift rotation problems:

- Stay as much as possible on a single shift.
- If you must work shift rotations, go with the clock, from days to evenings to nights.
- If you're on a permanent night-shift schedule, stick to a daily sleep routine during the day, even on your days off.
- If you know your shift change schedule, delay your bedtimes and rise times for 1 to 2 hours each night a few nights before your shift change.
- If you're scheduled on an on-call rotation (for example, if you're a physician), stay ahead of sleep debt with a regular sleep-wake schedule so you're as rested as possible before you start your on-call duties.
- For work, always try to find an area with increased light and sound at night.
- Bring a full-spectrum light bulb if possible.
- After a night shift, remember to wear sunglasses on your drive home to avoid sunlight cues.
- Experiment with phototherapy (see chapter 5) to help with rotating shifts.

- If you're a true "lark"—someone who wakes up early before an alarm with high energy in dawn and early morning hours, avoid night shift work. It's likely your system will struggle continuously.
- If you find it hard to sleep in the morning, when body temperature is rising, take advantage of the normal afternoon dip and sleep after lunch. Then try to take a quick postdinner nap to reduce your sleep debt.
- Protect your family life by letting children know when your shifts are and when they can expect you to be more available during the day.
- Keep in good communication with your spouse and children by leaving notes and carrying a pager and cell phone. Timed check-in calls make everyone feel more secure.

~ TOP SLEEP STEALERS FOR WOMEN ~

Organic illness (includes mood disorders)

Caffeine, alcohol, nicotine

Anxiety and/or chronic stress

Irregular sleep-wake schedule

Sub-clinical depression

Unresolved anger and/or resentments

Too much bedroom light, noise, poor air

Hidden food intolerances

Medication stimulant side effects

Extended napping

Hormonal changes or fluctuations

Calcium or magnesium deficiency

Pain

CHAPTER 8

IF YOU NEED
MORE HELP

ACUPUNCTURE

❧

How much bondage and suffering
a woman escapes when she takes the
liberty of being her own physician
of both body and soul.

—ELIZABETH CADY STANTON

IT'S ODD THAT ACUPUNCTURE IS STILL CONSIDERED an "alternative" therapy, considering that the East has practiced it for 2,500 years, and even now the esteemed National Institutes of Health declares, "The data in support of acupuncture are as strong as those for many accepted Western medical therapies." Insomnia is just one of scores of health conditions the World Health Organization lists as treatable by acupuncture.

Acupuncture's theory: Your body has an energy force—or *Qi* (pronounced "chee")—running through it, and your health is influenced by the flow or stagnation of your *Qi*. Free-flowing *Qi* means pink health, and blocked or trapped *Qi* means illness. Acupuncture also corrects your body's state of yin and yang energies. (In traditional Chinese medicine, *yin* is the natural feminine attributes of softness, darkness, receptiveness; *yang* is the male attributes of energy, movement, and light.)

Insomnia is seen as a deficient yin and an overactive yang condition. Acupuncture works by calming the central nervous system, balancing out the softer yin qualities while dampening the overactive yang.

How, briefly, does acupuncture work? An acupuncturist uses needles to stimulate any of the 365-or-so points along the fourteen primary body meridians or pathways through which Qi flows. This helps Qi flow back into balance and move to where it's deficient and away from where it's in excess. Needles vary in length, width of shaft, and shape of head, and an acupuncturist uses a few different, precise methods to insert the needles. Moxibustion, or the warming of the needles through certain herbs (usually powdered mugwort), also helps unblock Qi.

Science does not know how or why acupuncture works, but theories suggest that it stimulates secretions of endorphins (specifically Enkaphalins) and also helps balance neurotransmitter levels, such as serotonin and norepinephrine, both of which affect insomnia and disturbed sleep. It also boosts the immune system by raising levels of triglycerides, specific hormones, prostaglandins, white blood counts, gamma globulins, and overall antibody levels.

When looking for a good acupuncturist, remember a few things. Technique is important, and the skill of the acupuncturist is crucial, so do your homework. It's similar to finding a medical doctor, which many acupuncturists are, in TCM (Traditional Chinese Medicine) and in Western medicine. Your physician, local hospital, or TMC school may refer you; accreditation by the American Academy of Medical Acupuncturists is a plus. Check Resources for referral information in your area. Of course, personal referrals are best.

Make sure the acupuncturist uses disposable needles to prevent infection. Be sure to discuss any other treatments you are receiving; the acupuncturist should be able to tell you about possible interactions or aggravations of symptoms. Also, it's best if the acupuncturist informs your primary M.D. about your treatments so there is an open line of communication.

Generally, acupuncture is expensive; many health insurers don't yet cover treatments, or if they do, at only a fraction of the cost. And since acupuncture seems to work better for some people than others, you'll want to monitor your treatments carefully.

I remember the day I left the table after my first acupuncture treatment; I felt the endorphin-pumping effect for a full two days. As I kept up with treatments, my sleep pattern moved from erratic awakenings to a smooth, straight 6 hours. Give it a try, at least three or so sessions; you may well see a difference in your slumber.

HYPNOSIS

When the axe came into the forest,
the trees said the handle is one of us.
—TURKISH SAYING

HYPNOTHERAPY CONJURES UP SCARY IMAGES for people: subjects quacking like ducks, mad scientists, and seedy vaudeville stages. That's the entertainment use of hypnosis, which may or may not be real, and is certainly not therapeutic.

When hypnotherapy—the use of hypnosis for self-improvement and healing—is used as a medical adjunct, it's a potent mind-body technique that has backing by the very traditional National Institutes of Health (for chronic pain). It's real, and the trancelike state is not nearly as mysterious or Svengali-esque as portrayed.

Traditionally used by ancient Chinese and Egyptians, hypnotherapy today is practiced by many mainstream doctors (particularly anesthesiologists, surgeons, and, of course, psychiatrists), as well as a good number of dentists, psychotherapists, and nurses. It's often used for eliminating stubborn problem behaviors that appear resistant to other therapies. Insomnia is just one of the many symptoms hypnotherapy targets. (Weight loss, nicotine cessation, alcohol and drug addiction, chronic pain, phobias, panic attacks, and nightmares are a few others.)

Just how hypnosis works is scientifically debated, but it's accepted that the mind has two parts, the conscious and subconscious. During hypnosis, hypnotherapists help *facilitate* subjects to reach their subconscious mind by helping them fall into a trancelike state. If you haven't thought of trying hypnotherapy for your sleep troubles, give it some thought now. If you have prejudices and fears to overcome—and I had an ocean-full—good information is what you need most.

What will not happen when you undergo hypnosis: You will not be put under a "spell" or place yourself under the directive of someone who can transmute you into a murderess. You cannot be made to do something you don't want to do, and you'll probably feel fully alert and aware, though profoundly relaxed, during hypnosis, not a trivial experience in itself.

The process teaches you to exert control over your own behavior, emotions, subconscious mind, and what's stuck inside. Your choice of hypnotherapist is vital, so do your research carefully. A good idea is to get a referral from a friend or to find a medical professional who specializes in sleep issues and also works with hypnosis. (One caution: Anyone who suffers from a psychiatric illness must consult a physician, preferably a psychiatrist who is familiar with your condition.)

The hypnotic state isn't even that far-out once you experience it. If you've ever been dazed while listening to music, reading a book, driving, or creating in any capacity, you've experienced one type of hypnotic state, albeit a light one, termed a "superficial trance." The hypnotic alpha state is significantly deeper; here is where your heart rate, blood pressure, and respiration slow, and you're deeply relaxed. This is the stage used to eliminate problem behaviors like insomnia.

A deeper stage, mainly used by psychiatrists and psychotherapists, is sometimes termed "age regression" and helps reveal and heal painful memories that may be responsible for emotional and/or physical problems.

Remember, in order for hypnosis to work effectively, you must be fully willing to be hypnotized, you need to both trust and to have a positive relationship with your therapist, and you must be open to what hypnotism can do for you. Your hypnotherapist gives you some kind of technique or "anchor"—the touching of fingers, say—to help you slip into the highly relaxed trance state outside the therapy room. The consistent practice of this self-hypnosis anchor is also important if you're to keep positive results stable.

Personally, I was so afraid of hypnosis, for a variety of reasons, it took me three tribunal-like sessions with my therapist to get all my questions and misunderstandings assuaged. However, once I had all the information I needed, I opened a door to a rendezvous with unfinished subconscious business, one side effect of which was a long, fruitful period of longed-for, restful sleep.

CHIROPRACTIC CARE

*All sanity depends on this, that it
should be a delight to feel heat strike
the skin, a delight to stand upright,
knowing the bones are moving easily
under the flesh.*

—DORIS LESSING

MANY PEOPLE BELIEVE CHIROPRACTIC ADJUST-
ments help with pain, tension, fatigue, immunity,
strength, and even such things as asthma and migraine headaches. I've found that a wonderful side benefit of
regular chiropractic treatment is better, less fitful sleep.

Chiropractors see illness as stemming from a poorly
working spinal column. Poor posture, injury, disease, stressful
driving, hours spent sitting at a computer, a bad mattress and
sleeping positions, combined with a horde of other abuses,
configure to pull the spinal column off-kilter.

A good chiropractor adjusts—or manipulates—the
malfunctioning spinal areas, putting them back in strong
working order. My chiropractor adjusts with his hands what
I think is my fragile spine, using skilled and carefully directed
and controlled pressure and movements. I hear the familiar
"crack" and feel the pressure release, like a maypole in reverse.

I've noticed that when my neck and spine are out of
adjustment—when I've been lax about treatments or done

something to get my spine particularly out of whack—it shows up in my sleep. I'll wake up at odd intervals, almost as if there's a pressure point to my brain that needs to be turned off. And once the proper adjustments are done, in a few days, my sleep is improved.

To treat insomnia, chiropractic aims to desensitize the nerves on the spine. Think of it like a water hose: if you step on a small portion of it—impinging its flow—you still get water, just not a capacity amount. Since nerves rest on the outside of the spinal cord, the theory goes, when the subluxations or misalignments are corrected, the nerve flow up the spinal column is reopened and the insomnia problems lessen.

To determine if yours is a chiropractic candidate, take a good look at your lifestyle: Do you sit too much during the day at work, talk on the phone, overuse your back or leg muscles, run up and down stairs, move heavy products? Do you have neck, arm, leg, jaw, or upper or lower back pain? Pain medication can only do so much.

For work, I sit at a desk, use the telephone neck crunch endlessly, drive too much, sit and sleep in airplanes—all ripe for regular chiropractic twists. Thankfully, chiropractors are in the midst of a well-earned renascence, and I know many people who cling to their chiropractors like close friends.

If you've never tried chiropractic therapy, do. Done correctly, it can feel like someone's given rebirth to your spine. Many health insurance companies now pay for regular therapeutic visits, so use your benefits. It's a great way to get both your spine and your sleep straightened out.

BIOFEEDBACK

*The moment of change
is the only poem.*
−ADRIENNE RICH

BIOFEEDBACK IS WHAT YOU MIGHT IMAGINE:
feedback you get from a machine on your current
biological state. If you're tense and uptight, you will
see scientific proof, a somewhat unusual phenomenon when
it first occurs.

Used with great success for insomnia—particularly for
those insomniacs with highly tensed muscles—biofeedback
is an especially good treatment choice for sleep-troubled
women who experience headaches, migraines, or any other
chronic pain problems.

Using biofeedback, you learn to control your body's internal activities by monitoring them on a machine that uses
sound, light, or tone to give a play-by-play account of your
physiological state: your muscle tension, skin temperature,
blood pressure, heart rate, and a host of other pertinent bodily functions.

Biofeedback's theory: Once you become conscious of
normally occurring unconscious body functions, like breathing and muscle tension (the bio part), visual cues and sounds
via electronic devices (the feedback) help teach you to
change and control these physiological states, helping you

sleep better. EMG biofeedback, or electromyography, measures muscle tension and is the most commonly used insomnia treatment technique. Here, the monitor's electrodes attach to a muscle group identified as tense or painful and that's been keeping you awake.

For instance, your forehead muscles are strained. You're asked to consciously relax those muscles, which, at first, is a bit like being asked to wiggle your ears. Depending on the device, you'll get a tone signal or a beep, plus some sort of visual printout that changes along with your changing physiological state. If your muscles relax, you'll usually get a low tone. If you're not doing so well and tensing up, you'll hear a high tone.

In essence, the biofeedback machine trains you to produce the same muscle relaxation techniques whether you're lying in bed or hooked up to electrodes in an office. Gradually, you master what relaxed muscles actually feel like and what you must consciously do to get those muscles relaxed.

You can see how learning to relax one's body is a formative variable in any health equation—mental, physical, or spiritual. Most important, this helps you on your way to better rest.

Biofeedback is not the only muscle relaxation technique; there are other free self-relaxation techniques you can use in your own home. But if you have problems going it alone, try biofeedback. If it works, you've hit a gold mine. Once you've mastered the techniques, you take them with you, no need for costly repeat visits. (To find a biofeedback practitioner, see Resources for national network information.)

What was once seen as something of an oddity back in the '50s—a machine based on yogis and gurus who meditated their lowered blood pressures and tranced themselves into alpha wave stage 1 sleep—has now become a much-used sleep-repair tool. Who could have guessed?

ANY CODA TO A WOMAN'S SLEEP BOOK WOULD likely contain reference to visits by the Sandman and sleep fairies, as well as hopes and wishes for sweet sleep. Yes, may well-rested slumber meet you now and each and every time you lay your head on a pillow, close your eyes, and dream.

E quindi uscimmo a riveder le stelle.
And so we came forth, and once again beheld the stars.

ACKNOWLEDGMENTS & THANKS

To write this first book, I depended on the indulgence, guidance, love, understanding, endless conversations, and sustenance of many:

My parents, two Siamese jewels who absolutely adored being parents and who blessed and loved me in protective perfection. I could not have been loved anymore than by these two people, my heros.

My father's spirit, the kindest—and Lord knows rarest—of men, who bred and believed in this beautiful mind; he was a canopy for me under any hot sun. I still miss him every minute. What a gift he was, is, for a woman to carry with her all her life.

My mother, who poured herself into me and still does. If she but held my hand, I felt safe. You love me in incomprehensible ways. Merci à mama.

My brothers, whom I love; and with thanks to Kent, who has listened so much to my slumber worries. And to all the Max memories.

My nieces and nephews and all the wee ones to come. You will shake the world.

My fab colleagues who come and go and glow and come. All of you. Of all the plain and ordinary things you are not.

My Caretribe—my *amies,* you are my trophies of light. I am beyond rich in original friends. You help me breathe—

you keep me awake and teach me to keep out of my own way. I thank you for the sweet trust and the never-ended hearing. I love you. You know well who you all are.

My doctors. I have been blessed with extraordinary clinicians in my life, who have saved my life more times than I care to remember: Dr. Ellen Beauchamp, Susan Highleyman, and Dr. Robert Gerner.

All the thousands and thousands of interviewees in my career, who taught me to laugh, who taught me to think, who taught me how tiny and fragile we all are on this journey.

Ireland, ah, and all my heather friends, soil of my soul. You changed my life.

My unbidden angels at Conari: Leslie Berriman, and the rest. Thank you.

All sleep researchers, without whom.

The boys of ELJH, my huckleberry friends, you are Vikings.

The poets, who alone change the world.

My Aman Cara, who believed in me and believes me, and who made the waters part. You love me like the lily in the crook of God's arm.

The Redeemer; I love you even with my eyes closed.

All of you, who have loved me tender, this girl who looks so tame and so shy above this wild heart.

To the music of what happens.

RESOURCES

THE FOLLOWING ITEMS ARE FILLED WITH INFOR-
mation about all things sleep-related, from books
and music to help you sleep to national associations
and Internet Web sites. Enjoy the search.

~ BOOKS ~

Angier, Natalie. *Woman: An Intimate Geography.* New York: Houghton
Mifflin Co., 1999.

Beinfield, Harriet, and Korgold, Efrem. *Between Heaven and Earth: A
Guide to Chinese Medicine.* New York: Ballantine Books, 1992.

Benson, Herbert Dr. *The Relaxation Response.* New York: William
Morrow, 1975.

Bishop, Deborah, and Levy, David. *Hello Midnight: A Compendium to
Distract, Amuse, and Entertain the Dream Deprived.* New York:
Simon & Schuster, 2001.

Blate, Michael, and staff of G-Jo Institute. *Better Sleep with Acugenics.*
Davie, FL: Falkyn, Inc., for The G-Jo Institute, 1998.

Brown, Simon. *Practical Feng Shui.* London: Cassel & Co., 1997.

Casey, Nell. *Unholy Ghost: Writers on Depression.* New York: William
Morrow, 2001.

Chopra, Deepak. *Restful Sleep.* New York: Harmony Books, 1994.

Colbert, Don. *The Bible Cure for Sleep Disorders.* Orlando, FL: Siloam
Press, 1996.

Coren, Stanley. *Sleep Thieves: An Eye-Opening Exploration into the
Science and Mysteries of Sleep.* New York: The Free Press, 1996.

Davis, Courtney. *I Knew a Woman: The Experience of the Female Body.*
New York: Random House, 2001.

Dement, William C., and Vaughan, Christopher. *The Promise of Sleep.*
New York: Delacorte Press, 1999.

Dillard, Annie. *For the Time Being.* New York: Knopf, 1999.

Dillard, James, and Ziporyn, Terra. *Alternative Medicine for Dummies.* Foster City, CA: IDG Books Worldwide, 1998.

Dowing, George. *The Massage Book.* New York: Random House, 1972.

Dunkell, Samuel. *Goodbye Insomnia, Hello Sleep.* New York: Birch Lane Press, 1994.

Feltman, John. *Hands-On Healing.* Emmaus, PA: Rodale Press, 1989.

Fontana, David. *Teach Yourself to Dream.* San Francisco: Chronicle Books, 1997.

Gawain, Shakti. *Creative Visualization.* London and New York: Bantam, 1982.

George, Mike. *Learn to Relax: A Practical Guide to Easing Tension and Conquering Stress.* San Francisco: Chronicle Books, 1998.

Gleick, James. *Chaos: Making a New Science.* New York: Viking Penguin, 1987.

Goldberg, Philip, and Kaufman, Daniel. *Everybody's Guide to Natural Sleep.* Los Angeles: J. P. Tarcher, 1990.

Hauri, Peter, and Linde, Shirley. *No More Sleepless Nights.* New York: John Wiley & Sons, 1996.

Howard, Judy. *Bach Flower Remedies for Women.* London: The C. W. Daniel Company Ltd., 1997.

Huston, James E., and Lanka, Darlene. *Perimenopause: Changes in Women's Health After Thirty-five.* Oakland, CA: New Harbinger, 1997.

Jacobs, Gregg D. *Say Good Night to Insomnia.* New York: Henry Holt and Company, 1998.

Jamison, Kay Redfield. *An Unquiet Mind: A Memoir of Moods and Madness.* New York: Vintage Books, 1995.

Jouvet, Michel. Trans. by Laurence Garey. *The Paradox of Sleep: The Story of Dreaming.* Cambridge, MA: The MIT Press. 1999.

Kaptchuk, Ted J. *The Web That Has No Weaver: Understanding Chinese Medicine.* New York: McGraw Hill, 2001.

Katagiri, Dainin. *Returning to Silence.* Boston: Shambhala, 1998.

Keating, Thomas. *Open Mind, Open Heart: The Contemplative Dimension of the Gospel.* Rockport, MA: Element, Inc. 1991.

Kryger, Meir H., Roth, Thomas, and Dement, William C., Eds. *Principles and Practice of Sleep Medicine.* Philadelphia: W. B. Saunders Co., 2000.

Kuusisto, Stephen, Tall, Deborah, and Weiss, David. *The Poet's Notebook: Excerpts from the Notebooks of 26 American Poets.* New York: W. W. Norton & Company, 1995.

Lagatree, Kirsten M. *Feng Shui: Arranging Your Home to Change Your Life.* New York: Villard, 1996.

Lavie, Peretz. Trans. by Anthony Berris. *The Enchanted World of Sleep.* New Haven, CT: Yale University Press, 1996.

Lightman, Alan. *Einstein's Dreams.* New York: Warner Books, 1993.

Linn, Dennis, Fabricant Linn, Sheila, and Linn, Matthew. *Sleeping with Bread: Holding What Gives You Life.* New York: Paulist Press, 1995.

Maxwell-Hudson, Clare. *The Complete Book of Massage.* New York: Random House, 1988.

Merton, Thomas. *Day of a Stranger.* Salt Lake City: Gibbs M. Smith, 1981.

Morgan, David. *Sleep Secrets for Shift Workers and People with Off-Beat Schedules.* Duluth, MN: Whole Person Associates, 1996.

Muryn, Mary, and Spellman, Cathy Cash. *Water Magic: Healing Bath Recipes for the Body, Spirit, and Soul.* New York: Fireside, 1995.

Northrup, Christiane. *The Wisdom of Menopause: Creating Physical and Emotional Health and Healing During the Change.* New York: Bantam Doubleday Dell Publishing, 2001.

Reichman, Judith. *I'm Too Young to Get Old.* New York: Times Books, 1998.

Reps, Paul. *Zen Flesh, Zen Bones.* Boston: Shambhala, 1994.

Ross, Julia. *The Diet Cure.* New York: Penguin Books, 1999.

Roth, Gabrielle. *Sweat Your Prayers: Movement as Spiritual Practice.* New York: Penguin USA, 1999.

Shiller, David. *The Little Zen Companion*. New York: Workman Publishing, 1994.

Slavin, Sara. *The Art of the Bath*. San Francisco: Chronicle Books, 1997.

Thich Nhat Hanh. *The Miracle of Mindfulness*. Boston: Beacon Press, 1975.

Tomlinson, Cybèle. *Simple Yoga*. Berkeley, CA: Conari Press, 2000.

Vienne, Veronique. *The Art of Doing Nothing: Simple Ways to Make Time for Yourself*. New York: Clarkson Potter/Publishers, 1998.

Walsleben, Joyce A. and Baron-Faust, Rita. *A Woman's Guide to Sleep: Guaranteed Solutions for a Good Night's Rest*. New York: Crown Publishers, 2000.

Weil, Andrew. *Spontaneous Healing*. New York: Fawcett Columbine, 1995.

Wiedman, John. *Desperately Seeking Snoozin': The Insomnia Cure from Awake to ZZZZZ*. Memphis, TN: Towering Pines Press, 1999.

Wilson, Roberta. *Aromatherapy for Vibrant Health and Beauty*. New York: Avery Publishing Group, 1994.

Wolf, Naomi. *Misconceptions: Truth, Lies, and the Unexpected Journey into Motherhood*. New York: Doubleday, 2001.

Wolfson, Amy R. *The Woman's Book of Sleep: A Complete Resource Guide*. Oakland, CA: New Harbinger Publications, Inc., 2001.

Wuellner, Flora Slosson. *Prayer and Our Bodies*. Nashville, TN: The Upper Room, 1987.

Zammit, Gary K. *Good Nights: How to Stop Sleep Deprivation, Overcome Insomnia, and Get the Sleep You Need*. Kansas City: Andrews McMeel, 1997.

~ MUSIC FOR SLEEP ~

The American Boychoir. *The American Boychoir: Hymn*. Angel Records, 1995.

Anuna. *Anuna*. Celtic Heartbeat/Atlantic, 1993.

Bocelli, Andrea. *Cieli Di Toscana*. Sugar/Polydor, 2001.

Bocelli, Andrea. *Sacred Arias*. Phillips, 1999.

Callas, Maria. *Operatic Arias.* EMI Classics, 1986.

Chanticleer. *Chanticleer: Magnificat.* TelDec Classics International, 2000.

The Choir of Trinity College Cambridge, England. *Vocé.* Brentwood Music, 1987.

Choralschola Der Wiener Hoburgkapelle. *Gregorian Chant.* Phillips, 1985.

Compilation. *Cosmic Music: Meeting Angels Through Sound & Music.* Angel Records, 1997.

Einhorn, Richard, and Anonymous 4. *Voices of Light.* Sony Classical, 1994.

Elias, Jonathan. *The Prayer Cycle: Music for the Century.* Sony Classical, 1999.

ellipsis arts . . . *Celtic Lullaby.* ellipsis arts/The Relaxation Company, 1998.

Enya. *The Memory of Trees.* Reprise, 1995.

Jacobs, Shellie. *Echoes from the Catacombs.* Non-Perishable Music, 1995.

Jenkins, Karl. *Adiemus: Songs of Sanctuary.* Virgin Records America, 1995.

Lauridsen, Morten. *Lux Aeterna.* RCM, 1998.

McKennitt, Loreena. *The Book of Secrets.* Warner Bros., 1997.

McKennitt, Loreena. *A Winter's Garden.* Warner Bros., 1995.

Ni Riain, Noirin. *Soundings: Spiritual Songs from Many Traditions.* Sounds True Audio, 1995.

Project Ars Nova. *The Island of St. Hylarion: Music of Cypress.* New Albion Records, 1991.

Roth, Gabrielle. *Ritual.* Raven, 1995.

Sequentia. *Hildegard Von Bingen: Canticles of Ecstasy.* BMG Classics, 1994.

Shaw, Robert, and The Atlanta Symphony Orchestra & Chorus. *Choral Masterpieces.* Telarc, 1985.

Thompson, Jeffrey Dr. *Natural Music for Sleep, and Classical Music for Sleep.* Giama/The Relaxation Company, 2001.

~ ORGANIZATIONS ~

American Academy of Medical Acupuncturists
    AAMA
    1929 Wilshire Blvd., Suite 428
    Los Angeles, CA 90010
    (323) 937-5514
    aaa.medicalacupuncture.org

American Academy of Sleep Medicine
    6301 Bandel Rd., Suite 101
    Rochester, MN 55901
    (507) 287-6006; Fax: (507) 287-6008
    www.aasmnet.org

American Association of Retired Persons (AARP)
    601 E St., N.W.
    Washington, DC 20049
    (800) 424-3410
    www.aarp.org

American Association of Sex Educators,
    Counselors and Therapists
    P.O. Box 5488
    Richmond, VA 23220-0488
    AASECT@aasect.org

American Medical Women's Association
    801 N. Fairfax St., Suite 400
    Alexandria, VA 22314
    (708) 838-0500; Fax: (703) 549-3864
    www.amwa-doc.org

American Psychiatric Association
    1400 K St., N.W.
    Washington, DC 20005
    (800) 357-7924; (202) 682-6000; Fax: (202) 682-8650
    www.psych.org

American Psychological Association
    750 First St., N.E.
    Washington, DC 20002-4242
    (800) 374-2721; Fax: (202) 336-5500
    www.apa.org

American Sleep Apnea Association
    A.W.A.K.E. Network
    1424 K St., N.W., Suite 302
    Washington, DC 20005
    (202) 293-3650; Fax: (202) 293-3656
    www.sleepapnea.org

Anxiety Disorders Association of America
    11900 Parklawn Dr., Suite 100
    Rockville, MD 20852
    (301) 231-9350
    www.adaa.org

Arthritis Foundation
    P.O. Box 7669
    Atlanta, GA 30357-0669
    (800) 283-7800

Center for Narcolepsy
    Stanford University
    Sleep Disorders Research
    401 Quarry Rd., Room 3354
    Stanford, CA 94305
    (650) 725-6512
    www.med.stanford.edu

Depression After Delivery
    P. O. Box 278
    Belle Mead, NJ 08502
    (908) 575-9121

Fibromyalgia Network
    P. O. Box 31750
    Tuscon, AZ 85751-1750
    (800) 853-2929
    www.fmnetnews.com

The Lucidity Institute
    2555 Park Blvd., Suite 2
    Palo Alto, CA 94306-1919
    (800) GO-LUCID (465-8243); (650) 321-9969;
    Fax: (650) 321-9967
    www.lucidity.com

Migraine Awareness Group
    113 S. Saint Asaph, Suite 300
    Alexandria, VA 22314
    (703) 739-2432
    www.migraine.org

Narcolepsy Network
    Reed Hartman Corporate Center
    10921 Reed Hartman Highway
    Cincinnati, OH 45242
    (513) 891-3522; Fax: (513) 891-3836
    www.narcolepsynetwork.org

National Alliance for the Mentally Ill
    3 Colonial Place
    2107 Wilson Blvd., Suite 300
    Arlington, VA 22201-3042
    (702) 524-7600; (900) 950-NAMI; Fax: (703) 524-9094

National Asian Women's Health Organization
    250 Montgomery St., Suite 900
    San Francisco, CA 94101
    (415) 989-9747; Fax: (415) 989-9758
    www.nawho.org

National Black Women's Health Project
    1237 Ralph David Abernathy Blvd., S.W.
    Atlanta, GA 30310
    (404) 758-9590

National Center on Sleep Disorders Research
    Two Rockledge Center, Suite 7024
    6701 Rocklede Dr., MSC 7920
    Bethesda, MD 20892-7920
    (301) 435-0199; Fax: (301) 480-3451
    www.nhlbi.nih.gov

National Depressive and Manic-Depressive Association
   730 N. Franklin St., Suite 501
   Chicago, IL 60610-7204
   (800) 826-3632; Fax: (312) 642-7243
   www.ndmda.org

National Headache Foundation
   428 W. Saint James Pl., 2nd Floor
   Chicago, IL 60614-2750
   (888) NHF-5552; Headache hotline (800) 843-2256;
   (773) 288-6399; Fax: (773) 525-7357
   www.headaches.org

National Institutes of Mental Health
   NIMH Public Inquires
   6001 Executive Blvd., Room 8184, MSC 9663
   Bethesda, MD 20892-9663
   (301) 443-4513; Fax: (310) 443-4279
   www.nimh.nih.gov

National Latina Health Organization
   P. O. Box 7567
   Oakland, CA 94601
   (510) 534-1362

National Lesbian and Gay Health Association
   Lesbian Health Advocacy Network
   1407 S St., N.W.
   Washington, DC 20009
   (202) 797-3536

National Mental Health Information Center
   1020 Prince St.
   Alexandria, VA 23314-2971
   (800) 969-6642

National Sleep Foundation
   1522 K St., N.W., Suite 500
   Washington, CD 20005
   (202) 341-3471; Fax: (202) 341-3472
   www.sleepfoundation.org

North American Menopause Society
  P. O. Box 94527
  Cleveland, OH 44101-4527
  (440) 442-7550; Fax: (440) 442-2660
  www.menopause.org

Postpartum Support International
  927 N. Kellogg Ave.
  Santa Barbara, CA 93111
  (805) 967-7636; Fax: (805) 967-0608
  www.postpartum.net

Restless Legs Syndrome Foundation
  819 Second St., S.W.
  Rochester, MN 55902-2985
  www.rls.org

Sex Information and Education Council of the U.S.
  30 W. 42nd St., Suite 350
  New York, NY 10036
  (212) 819-9770; Fax: (212) 819-9776
  www.siecus.org

Society for Light Treatment and Biological Rhythms
  P. O. Box 591687
  174 Cook St.
  San Francisco, CA 94159-1687
  Fax: (415) 751-2758
  www.sltbr.org

World Federation of Sleep Research Societies
  c/o Michael Chase, Ph.D.
  Brain Research Institute, UCLA School of Medicine
  Center for the Health Sciences
  43-367
  Los Angeles, CA 90095-1746
  (310) 825-3417; Fax: (310) 206-3499
  www. wfsrs.org

~ WEB SITES ~

American Sleep Disorders Association (ASDA) Home Page
www.asda.org

A.P.N.E.A. Net
www.apneanet.org

The Association for the Study of Dreams
www.asdreams.org

BabyCenter
www.babycenter.com/pregnancysleep

Biofeedback Network
www.biofeedback.net

Endometriosis.org
www.endometriosis.org

Menopause Online
www.menopause-online.com

The Mid-Life and Menopause Support Group
www.span.com.au/midlife/index.html

PeriodWatch.com
www.periodwatch.com

Sleep Medicine Home Page
www.users.cloud9.net/~thorpy

SleepNet
www.sleepnet.com

Sleep Support Group
alt.support.sleep-disorder

The Sleep Well
Stanford/Dr. William Dement
www.stanford.edu/~dement

Talk about Sleep
www.talkaboutsleep.org

UCLA's Sleep Home Pages
Brain Information Service
bisleep.medsch.ucla.edu

0304

ABOUT THE AUTHOR

J ANET KINOSIAN IS AN AWARD-WINNING JOURNALIST who has written for the *Los Angeles Times, Los Angeles Times Magazine, Washington Post, W, Saturday Evening Post,* and *Reader's Digest,* among many others. She has a B.A. in Psychology from UCLA and an M.A. in Counseling Psychology from Loyola Marymount University. She did postgraduate studies in poetry and creative writing at Harvard University and has won a New Letters Poetry Prize. She lives and sleeps near Los Angeles, California. Her immediate goal is to become a champion sleeper.

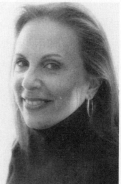

photo by Levon Parian

For more information about Janet and her work, visit her Web site at http://www.wellrestedwoman.com.